COMPASSIONATE ACTIVISM

COMPASSIONATE ACTIVISM

An Exploration of Integral Social Care

Mark Garavan

PETER LANG

Oxford · Bern · Berlin · Bruxelles · Frankfurt am Main · New York · Wien

Bibliographic information published by Die Deutsche Nationalbibliothek
Die Deutsche Nationalbibliothek lists this publication in the Deutsche Nationalbibliografie;
detailed bibliographic data is available on the Internet at http://dnb.d-nb.de.

A catalogue record for this book is available from the British Library.

Library of Congress Cataloging-in-Publication Data:

Garavan, Mark, 1965-
  Compassionate activism : an exploration of integral social care / Mark
Garavan.
     p. cm.
  Includes bibliographical references and index.
  ISBN 978-3-0343-0848-9 (alk. paper)
  1. Social service. 2. Caregivers. 3. Caring. I. Title.
  HV40.G363 2012
  361.2--dc23

                         2012008373

ISBN 978-3-0343-0848-9

Peter Lang AG, International Academic Publishers, Bern 2012
Hochfeldstrasse 32, CH-3012 Bern, Switzerland
info@peterlang.com, www.peterlang.com, www.peterlang.net

Printed in Germany

Contents

Foreword

The immediate cause for writing this book has been my participation in developing and lecturing on a degree programme in Applied Social Studies. The book is a response to the challenges and issues raised in being obliged to think from first principles about contemporary social care both as a professional practice and as a task for all citizens. The ideas set out here therefore are the result not only of my academic and social care work experiences over a twenty-five-year period but from an engagement with a large number of students in more recent years. Many of these students were highly experienced social care practitioners in their own right. All, whether new to the field or otherwise, have enriched my understanding of the issues that are addressed herein. This book could not have been written without them and for that I am deeply grateful.

I dedicate this book to the memory of Frank O'Leary, a true exemplar of compassionate activism. Frank was a founding member of the Dublin Simon Community. He died in 1989 just as Simon was occupying its new, purpose-built emergency night shelter on Usher's Island in Dublin. He left behind great numbers of friends and colleagues forever inspired by his commitment and care. I count myself as one of those.

PART ONE

What is Care?

Introduction

The term 'social care' is one that we are familiar with. We use it to designate a wide range of intentional, paid and formal social interactions such as in childcare, youth work, work with people with physical and intellectual disabilities, work with prisoners, drug addicts, asylum seekers and the elderly. Social care seems to be all around us and to encompass a very wide range of activities. Most of us at some time have probably received, or known someone who has received, formal social care. Yet, even though it seems so widespread, have we seriously thought about what social care is meant to be? Have we rigorously considered what it is that we are trying to achieve by social care? What precisely are we doing when we do social care? And is social care an activity only for paid practitioners? Do we really need to pay somebody to care?

This book sets out to try and address these questions. We appear to be at an opportune moment to think about such matters. First, at the present time, formal social care in Ireland is undergoing a transition into professionalism. Under the Health and Social Care Professionals Act 2005, a registration system is being proposed which will legally designate the boundaries and standards of the new profession according to prescribed education and training criteria. As a result, new national guidelines for Third Level education providers have been drawn up by the Higher Education and Training Awards Council. But, despite this movement towards regulation, is social care as a concept and practice fully understood? Do we have an adequate theoretical conception of what social care is and what its purposes are? Have we, as part of this journey to professionalism, whether we are educators, practitioners or receivers of 'care', engaged in a rigorous reflection on the assumptions underlying social care?

Second, the last number of years in Ireland has seen a series of truly shocking reports containing revelations into the standards and conditions pertaining in formal, institutional care settings. The most appalling has certainly been the *Ryan Report*, which found that there was systematic abuse in our traditional church-run childcare institutions of reformatory and industrial schools. Nothing can be, or should be, the same after the *Ryan Report*. It revealed how an entire apparatus of care, purportedly designed to cherish and nurture children, became utterly dysfunctional due to warped ideologies, abusive practices by some and a pervasive moral cowardice by many which led to widespread *de facto* collusion. But there has also been the report of the Leas Cross Nursing Home Enquiry, the report on the death of Tracey Fay, reports on other deaths of children in State care and many others, such as the *Roscommon Childcare Case Report*. Our treatment of prisoners, particularly in Mountjoy Prison, of people with physical disability and of asylum seekers in our direct provision hostels is nothing short of scandalous.[1] People continue to die in Ireland due to neglect and deprivation.[2] The cumulative effect of all of these revelations has been to bring into question precisely what we are doing in our system of care.[3]

Thus, formal social care practice at present seems particularly undermined and its claims, both theoretical and empirical, to be 'person-centred' appear suspect. In this fraught context, it seems helpful to go back to

---

1   See for example the annual reports of the Mountjoy Prison Visiting Committee, the 2010 report of the Working Group on People with Physical Disabilities in 'Congregated Settings', FLAC's 2009 report into direct provision accommodation, *One Size Doesn't Fit All*, and Amnesty International's 2011 report *In Plain Sight*.

2   In the ten years from 2000 to 2009 almost 200 children died while either in State care or while known to State care services. In the same period, forty-eight people died in Direct Provision hostels due to a variety of causes. As we shall note below, the Health Research Board has found that as many as 5,400 people die annually in Ireland due to poverty and inequality.

3   Such concerns are not, of course, confined to Ireland. For example, in a letter published in *The Telegraph* newspaper in January 2012 more than sixty UK government advisors, charity directors and independent experts described England's social care system as failing, leaving 800,000 elderly people 'lonely, isolated and at risk'.

basics. What is social care? What does it seek to achieve and how does it get there? I hope that this book will be a contribution to answering these crucial questions.

The ideas contained in this book serve a dual purpose. On the one hand, they may be helpful in examining and reflecting upon what contemporary professional social care might involve. The book will describe professional practice as a liberating, ethically framed relationship with another person that should give rise to an exciting project of mutual humanization. Yet, on the other hand, a core argument of the book will be that social care is about far more than professional practice. Quite apart from the reality that there are vast numbers of domestic 'carers' directly looking after loved ones at home and that informal caring is a ubiquitous feature of human behaviour, a commitment to social care is an issue for everybody in society. This is so in the sense that all of us, as citizens and members of a society, should be engaged in a concern with, and a commitment to, the well-being of all who share our social world. The specific reasons as to why this might be the case are treated in detail in later chapters. Therefore, right at the outset, I want to claim that we need to expand what we understand by the term 'social care' and that the theoretical content of 'social care' is about far more than training a corps of professional practitioners. In short, social care is not just a demarcated professional practice but rather is an activity for everyone.

In fact, I believe that considering how we might all become 'social carers' offers us a valuable and helpful way to re-imagine our relationships with each other, with our societies and, even more ambitiously, with the earth and wider earth community. This broader commitment to, and expanded understanding of, social care, I will designate as 'compassionate activism'. My view is that compassionate activism offers us a way to be fully human and certainly is a more fulfilling and beneficial way than that offered by the multitude of 'self-help' and 'self-improvement' books and manuals that promise happiness and serenity in easy steps.

Caring for the whole person

The verb 'to care' can carry a somewhat patronizing aura. Caring for someone seems to evoke images of helping, of charity, of mercy, of pity and of
attempting to make up for someone else's deficits or disabilities. It appears
to assume a relationship exchange that involves a giver and a receiver and
a clear distinction between which person is which. It suggests a relationship initiated by a visible need on the part of one person and a meeting
of that need on the part of the other. In the case of Ireland, the historical
origin of much of our social care activity within Christian religious 'works
of mercy' and the Victorian Poor Law system may further reinforce this
ethos of deficit and charity.

This is one of the reasons why I propose that the term compassionate
activism better captures the dynamic, interactional and developmental
character of integral social care engagement. Of course, simply substituting
a term does not necessarily change an empirical reality. Much contemporary care work may well continue to draw from charitable motivations. In
a Western cultural context still centred largely on the individual and still
ideologically averse to understanding human beings in socio-structural
terms, nineteenth-century conceptions of what constitutes social care
practice remain potent.

Indeed, it must be recognized that many people (certainly, initially
at least, many students who wish to be practitioners) if asked to define
social care are likely to describe it in terms of an interpersonal interaction
between a knowledgeable, albeit considerate, helping subject and a visibly
needy, albeit deserving, receiving object. The skills therefore adjudged to
better enable this interaction to succeed concentrate on communication,
evaluation and relevant technical and practical competencies.

These skills of course are of profound importance. But, if they are
regarded as the only, or primary, skills involved in social care then, I believe,
we have made a fundamental conceptual error. Social care cannot pay attention only to the interpersonal interaction and cannot assume a simple and
clear demarcation between 'carers' and the 'cared-for'. For that reason, a

second key argument to be made in this book is that genuinely committed social care, i.e. social care designed to be fully effective, involves the practitioner-citizen operating in two complementary dimensions. The first is indeed the interpersonal dimension. The second however is the dimension of the political and social. Thus, *integral social care* is care that addresses and responds to the individual in both their interpersonal dynamic and settings and in their wider socio-political dynamics and settings. In short, the compassionate activist, in order to comprehensively care for the person before him/her, combines caring and campaigning.

This may seem at first sight like an unnecessary and indeed unwelcome extension of the practice of social care. Conventionally, it appears that our understandings of social care tend to exclusively concentrate on the personal but are less liable to include the political. There are a number of possible explanations for this. The most obvious is likely to be that care – as a visible human expression and behaviour – is indeed made most manifest and is most experienced at the interpersonal level. Smiling, touching and listening are inherently interpersonal actions. These are gestures that we can all accomplish and can see the immediate benefit of. But the circumstances of need and suffering that people find themselves in may be the result of wider social processes. Fully resolving their situation may therefore require addressing these wider causes. To summarize it briefly, the cause and resolution of someone's grief and problems may lie not within their own private competence but within wider socio-political processes. In addition, the decisions and circumstances determining those who we personally are likely to encounter, those who we define as formally in need of receiving care and those who we regard as worthy of our care are likely to be the result not only of our own personal decisions but of wider sociological factors beyond our control.

Thus, integral social care must be attentive to both these dimensions of the person. Social care, to be effective, must include both the personal and the political. The interplay between the two dimensions is of course highly complex. However, in order to recognize the connection between them, we need to think not only beyond our natural orientation towards the personal domain, we may also be obliged to overcome a more general but very powerful, ideologically created assumption about human beings.

This assumption is that of the autonomous self-interested individual. The autonomous, rational actor is the ideal-type human of the Western world. This individual is understood to be the author of their own biography and master of their own life. They are responsible for their own social well-being. Success or failure is regarded as largely their own responsibility. They are accountable for their own actions. They are meant to know what they want, who they are, what they are doing and what it is that they want to achieve.

This radical individualism, which has become more prominent in the last few decades with the re-emergence of conservative and neo-liberal ideas, has had significant implications in shaping social care work and theory and in determining welfare policies and practices. If the practitioner-citizen subscribes to this conception of the individual, then the focus of care should consequently be on encouraging the subject to become an autonomous rational actor in line with the norm. Welfare or care 'dependency' should be avoided so, on that basis, the quicker the subject takes charge of their own life the better. The success or failure of that life will therefore ultimately indeed be their own responsibility.

The difficulty however is that this notion of the autonomous individual is largely an ideological myth. It is the product of high modernity, bequeathed to us in part by the philosopher Descartes but reaching its intellectual culmination in Liberalism. As we shall see later on in this book, it is of fundamental importance that we achieve a correct and balanced understanding of the human person. The fact is that human beings are the product of incredibly complex sociological, biological and psychological *processes* and *structures*. They are not created *de novo*. Nor can they possibly ever inhabit or live within an asocial or non-culturally conditioned setting. Each individual is always implicated in the fate of all. In the same way that biological evolution shapes our physical structure so too does culture (understood as our entire way of life) indelibly shape our social and psychological structure.

In short, to understand any human individual involves understanding them not just as unique persons but also understanding the entire complex matrix of cultural, social, historical and political forces which have shaped them. Supporting effective change for any individual can therefore be seen as involving not just a transforming of their personal attributes and attitudes but also engaging with the entire contextual structure of forces which constitutes their identity and constrains their social freedom.

There are thus always these two dimensions to the human person to be considered – the personal/interpersonal and the social/political. Integral social care must address both. However, recognizing these domains means not just overcoming the myth of the autonomous self-interested individual but also the myth of society as somehow 'natural' and grounded on an unchanging understanding of 'human nature'. This latter idea suggests that society is fixed, is as it is because it could not be in any other way. In fact, when viewed historically, human societies and cultures are incredibly varied and malleable. They are constructed according to certain key and identifiable forces which are often economic and ideological/religious in character. As they are constructed so they can be reconstructed. That societies are subject to the possibility of change and are, in fact, continually changing permits us to raise the question of what kind of change should there be. Who should it favour? Who determines and directs such changes? Can it be change which increases integral social care or decreases it?

Thus, a more holistic conception of the human person must include both personal and social dimensions. The truth of the matter is that we are neither fully autonomous nor fully conditioned. We exist within a tension between these two poles. Human social behaviour is driven by two fundamental concerns. On the one hand, we want to belong. Belonging is a biological and cultural necessity. To be human we must be part of a tribe, a social-familial band, a society. Hence, our drive to belong causes us to share the same language, the same accents, the same tastes, the same values and beliefs, the same standards of behaviour, etiquette and manners as others in our group. Just watch any band of young people today and see how they unwittingly mimic each other, however unconsciously, down to the smallest details.

However, on the other hand we want to be truly ourselves. We want to be unique. We want to live our own lives, make our own choices and express our own views. Sometimes, as we each know from our personal experience, our desire to be ourselves conflicts with our desire to belong. This tension may give rise to great suffering (forming much of the substance of our psychological dramas and traumas) but also great creativity. This theme of how we become a full and liberated person is one that we shall return to continually in this book.

The relevance of all of these preliminary observations is based on the recognition that the subject and object of integral social care is the human being. Engaging with human beings is always an ethical endeavour and one implication of this is that we have a sound and secure grasp of who we are dealing with. The point is that if we have a reductionist or overly individualized understanding of human problems then we shall fail to adequately and competently bring about integral social care.

In this sense a core value and concern of integral social care must be effectiveness. Are we truly humanizing and liberating ourselves and those with whom we work? Our own positive mental or emotional disposition towards the other person is important of course but integral social care relationships should primarily be about the humanization and the liberation of the other person not about whether we feel good or wanted in providing that care. Our emotions and positive regard for others may fluctuate but our effectiveness should not.

Purpose of care

This concern to be effective in turn raises the question posed above of what it is we are striving to achieve. How precisely do you measure and attain humanization and liberation? What does it really look like? This is a question of the utmost importance and is one that will lie at the heart of this book. To start with, we need to consider whether our goal is the 'normalizing' of someone or the 'integration' of someone into the social mainstream. These are inelegant terms, laden with value judgements and assumptions. After all, what if the social norm could itself be regarded as dysfunctional and unjust? Is being 'average' really the apex of being human?

These questions will be returned to throughout this book. They warrant considered attention. Of great importance in addressing this issue will be the third core argument of the book which is that authentic compassionate activism involves us in an exhilarating dynamic that leads to our own humanization. We will explore further on what we might mean by humanization but, for now, let us tentatively suggests that it involves the person becoming free to become who they want to be through a process of discovery encountered in the exercise of making free choices. This definition rests in turn on the assumption that human beings are not fixed and complete but are always, through their choices, forging their own identity. It will also be suggested that the direction of that process of discovery, in order to expand the person's deepest human potential and capabilities, is best achieved through experiencing and practising our deep intrinsic capacities of care and compassion. If this is so, then one can validly argue that deep and respectful engagement with each other can enhance our humanity and deliver a truer, more fulfilling version of ourselves. For this reason, integral and caring relationships constitute a privileged path to the attainment of our own humanity.

This is so both for 'carer' and those being 'cared for'. Indeed, we need to be cautious about assuming that there is a clear distinction to be made between care-givers and care-receivers. The truth is that in our journey through life each of us at different times may be carers and recipients of care. We can expect to occupy both positions at some time. In addition, much care-giving is done by those who themselves simultaneously are receiving care. This is particularly true for many women throughout the world. The mutual enrichment involved in giving and receiving care, attested to by so many who are engaged in integral social care, professionally or otherwise, can lead us out of our incredibly narrow contemporary conception of what it is to be human, a conception of us as self-interested, rational actors primarily concerned with maximizing our own utility. This deeply constrained vision of ourselves – clearly empirically false – has led us into grave dysfunctions and unhappiness. This is an assertion that will be treated and supported in the next chapter.

In summary, the great purpose of compassionate activism, why we should embrace it, is that it leads not only to the enhancement of others but leads to our own humanization as well. If this mutuality is not present then this is a sure sign that the version of care being deployed is false and oppressive. However, let us concede openly that there is no compelling proof in favour of this understanding of humanization. All one can ultimately say is that *if* we can become more human through integral relationships – more caring, more compassionate, both personally and socially – then we *ought* to do so. This book tries to explore how this can be done and why it should be done.

Thus, compassionate activism (as a way to re-imagine integral social care) can be conceptualized as a project to achieve humanization which in turn is understood as involving personal and social liberation. Compassionate activists, conscious of their own limitations, enter into relationships with people who suffer some form of oppression and constraint, yet who are full of capacity and capability, in order to *mutually and effectively* liberate each other. In so far as training is required for those who wish to be professional integral social carers it should concentrate on the two important domains highlighted above: interpersonal skills which focus on authenticity, effectiveness and acceptance of the other person, and socio-political skills which focus on developing a critical consciousness and understanding of social structures and changes. For this reason, Parts Two and Three of this book address each of these areas in turn.

However, as indicated already, this book is not a training manual for professional carers. It does not purport to be a definitive account of contemporary issues in social care. There are many challenges in contemporary social care practice which are not addressed comprehensively here – law and legal issues, resources, work practices, management capabilities and staff supports. These various matters are examined in other texts and dealt with there far more comprehensively than this book could attempt.[4] Rather, this book is an exploration of some of those deeper theoretical and practical

---

4   See, for example, Perry Share and Kevin Lalor (2009), *Applied Social Care – An Introduction for Irish Students*, Dublin: Gill & Macmillan. See also Celesta McCann James *et al* (2009), *Social Care Practice in Ireland – an integrated perspective*, Dublin: Gill & Macmillan.

issues which I believe warrant specific notice and which draw our attention to the wider implications – both personal and social – of what we really might mean in committing ourselves to integral social care.

The book will proceed by arguing that care is a fundamental disposition and orientation of the human being. The empirical evidence shows that rather than being self-interested rational actors, human beings are far more likely to be compassionate and concerned for the welfare of others. The two domains of our compassionate activism will then be examined by paying particular attention to the work and thought of Carl Rogers and Paulo Freire. Rogers' ideas provide rich insights into the domain of the interpersonal and have given rise to some of the most basic values and orientations guiding person-centred therapeutic relationships, such as 'non-judgemental acceptance' and congruence. Freire's work offers a valuable framework to conceptualize both the process and goal of humanization in the social and political spheres. His work lays particular emphasis on the significance of dialogue in achieving personal and social transformation. Both have in common a deep humanism, one that can accommodate diverse sets of beliefs and values around a common, fundamental commitment to the integral liberation of the human being.

In my view there can be nothing more important than identifying this as the purpose of integral care. The human person in all their dignity and depth is the goal, subject and object of social care. This may seem either like a cliché or a truism but in this book I want to explore this wider and richer dimension to our commitment and the real implications of that commitment, precisely so that it is not reduced to a cliché. That is why I will argue that such a commitment raises issues not just for professional practitioners but for all who want to bring about a more human, more just and more ecological world.

I have used the term compassionate activism to capture this more holistic and inclusive conception of social care. No doubt, other terms could equally be selected. To fill out the content of this integral activism, the book examines in Part Two the interpersonal dimension of care and in Part Three the socio-political aspects. The characteristics and demands of each are analysed in detail. The book concludes in Part Four by proposing possible applications of this integral understanding of care and particularly how we might re-model our formal service structure. It will be suggested that the term 'dialogic practice' best describes the methods to be used in integral social care. Indeed, it will be argued that dialogue, both as a method and an ethic, is central to the process of humanization and offers us a readily available way to achieve interpersonal and socio-political change. Finally, the book tries to show how the commitment to care is rooted in a fundamental ethical orientation towards human well-being and welfare and what this means in practical terms for social care practice.

In this sense at least, this book is not neutral. It takes a stance and argues for a specific and particular personal and social vision of integral care. This vision is centred on a commitment to human freedom and a consequent opposition to all systems that repress that freedom. Therefore, it takes the position of those who suffer, either due to personal or to social factors, and which causes them to be socially excluded or marginalized. Adopting this position involves us in shifting our perspective to those who are 'below' – those on the underside of our society. This epistemological and methodological perspective reveals the social world in a new light, one which allows us to judge, interpret and assess social reality from a new viewpoint – that of the oppressed. Thus we pose new generating questions such as

- What does this society / world look like from the perspective of the poor and excluded?
- How do we judge this society from the perspective of the poor and excluded?

The reason for adopting this position is that the excluded human beings among us provide a clear and empirical measure of 'progress' or 'development'. Their very existence cuts through the simulated forms of constructed reality which enshroud and delude so many of us. By their existence, they challenge us to make real our commitment to solidarity and justice. They also shame us of course and can evoke in us the necessary compassion to recognize that our abundance and ease is frequently grounded on their exclusion and oppression.

The message of this book (if we can speak of 'message') is one of hope. Our commitment to each other and especially to the suffering and marginalized among us, not only restores those whom we encounter to their humanity, it also restores us to ours. This is the great paradox and joy of compassionate activism. In giving we truly do receive. In seeking to treat all others as fully human, we render ourselves as fully human as well. In this way, integral social care is the very foundation of what we can regard as civilization. A civilized society is one grounded on a culture of care.

Finally, for clarity, a brief concluding word on nomenclature. I refer to integral social care to mean care focused on the interpersonal and socio-political aspects of the human person. I use this term to include professional practitioners and committed citizens alike. Where there is a distinction to be drawn between them I make that clear as appropriate. I employ the term compassionate activism to describe the spirit, values and praxis that should inform integral care. In speaking of those who are the recipients of care, I use the terms the 'poor' or the 'oppressed'. These terms encompass those who are receiving formal or institutional social care services and those who are not. I do so aware that these are loaded terms. By poor I mean those who cannot mobilize resources in the way the non-poor can. Such resources may be either material such as money or shelter, or they may be symbolic such as language ability or outward signs of 'normality'. By oppressed I mean those whose freedom to be themselves has been constrained or limited by personal or social factors. These are deliberately provocative terms because I wish that we are disturbed by the reality that they refer to. I hope that their use will be justified by the treatment of the issues undertaken throughout this book.

The practice of social care is of course ubiquitous and therefore we need to recognize that it is not solely confined to an exchange between the 'non-poor' and the 'poor'. On the contrary, the most effective forms of care are often those practised among those who themselves share similar challenges and constraints. Many primary carers in many societies, women especially, are themselves excluded and marginalized. In addition, as noted above, we need to always acknowledge that each of us find ourselves in our lives on a continuum between caring and receiving, between capability and need.

CHAPTER TWO

Why Should We Care?

What kind of creature is the human being? Are we spiritual souls trapped in material bodies longing for redemption? Or are we hapless vehicles for selfish genes determined only on their own reproduction? Are we inherently good or bad, altruistic or selfish, rational or irrational? Do we occupy some strange unsettling place famously halfway between worm and God?

Almost certainly right from the beginning of human culture, small social bands and tribes have told each other stories that attempt to answer these types of profound questions. Such stories are constructed and framed according to each culture's own understandings and puzzlements about the world.[1] Not only do these stories provide explanatory frameworks within which we discover origin accounts about ourselves and answers about who we are, these accounts in turn shape our very behaviour itself. We enact these stories in our actions. In other words, the manner in which we conceptualize what human beings are in turn shapes the very way in which we experience being human.

The Indian brave on a spirit quest; the aborigine walking through a dreamtime landscape; the Japanese kamikaze pilot; the medieval Christian penitent walking barefoot to Rome; the Tibetan lama meditating in a cave for decades; the consumer striding through a shopping mall; all of these are images of human beings but are images rooted within quite specific cultural frameworks which provide the scale of values and meaning which render these activities purposeful, rational and honourable.

Our *picture* of being human shapes *how* we are human. Therefore the manner in which we conceptualize humanity and humanization is of critical

---

1   See Berry, Thomas (1988), *The Dream of the Earth*, San Francisco: Sierra Club Books.

importance. The sheer incredible diversity of human cultures across space and time demonstrates the extraordinary extent to which human beings differ. Some cultures accord status to having elongated necks. Others accord status to looped ear lobes. Others again to tiny feet. Some value material accumulation but others value giving everything away in an annual potlatch. Some cultures accord status to those who are brave in battle. Others value life so much they sweep the ground before taking each step. Some cultures believe that there are spirits in the plants and animals, others that there is one god dwelling in the sky. What each culture gives status to indicates what it values, and what it values sets out in turn what its standard is for good human behaviour.

Of course, given our long biological evolution, there are many fundamental common bahaviours and values to be found in all cultures. The wonderful American science fiction writer Kim Stanley Robinson outlined a number of these in his novel *Fifty Degrees Below* (2006: 127–8):

- Talking – vocalizations
- Walking upright – (down from the trees to the savannah)
- Running
- Dancing
- Singing
- Stalking animals
- Throwing things at things
- Looking at fire
- Having sex
- Dealing with the opposite sex more generally
- Cooking and eating the Paleolithic diet
- Gathering plants to eat
- Killing animals for food
- Experiencing terror

What is particularly striking about human beings however is that if we take the two most fundamentally biological behaviours – feeding and reproduction – we find that human cultures construct rules and conventions that temper and socialize these behaviours. Thus feeding, rather than being an anarchic frenzy of aggression where the strongest eats most and hoards all that he/she can, becomes instead a primordial social activity where food is shared and distributed. While this is frequently in accordance with status hierarchies (those with high status eat first and eat most) nonetheless the sharing of food ensures that the young, the old and the sick are nurtured and included. Indeed, communal eating may lie at the very roots of our sociality and be a key locus in the ongoing development of social bonding, communication and ultimately language. In a similar way, sex is regulated and managed within cultural groups so that rules and taboos emerge which socialize this potentially disruptive drive. Status hierarchies, courtship rituals and moral conventions all develop to regulate and discipline so powerfully biological a force as sexuality.

Even today, within micro-social settings, grabbing food and stuffing as much of it into your mouth before anyone else eats would constitute a grave social offence. The same is true of course for rape and sexual assault. Interestingly, it can be observed that courtship rituals (even contemporary ones) and shared eating are closely linked. How we eat may reveal much about our wider social commitment and integration. Thus, if we pursue this observation into modern times, we could speculate that today's Western eating pattern of individualized 'grazing' of fast food and microwaved pre-prepared meals may indeed show much regarding the character of modern social relations. In addition, Western over-consumption of food and the configuration of the food consumed, particularly the quantity of meat, when contrasted with wider global patterns of hunger and malnutrition, further underlines the social significance and meaning of how we eat.[2]

The primary point however to be made here is that human culture socializes biology. How this socialization occurs and the values and objectives which inform it reveals to us the essential character of the particular culture concerned. In this context, it is clear why that culture's dominant understanding of what it is to be human is of such importance. The ideal

2   See, for example, C. Petrini and G. Padovanni (2006), *Slow Food Revolution: A New Culture for Dining and Living*, New York: Rizzoli International.

model the culture has of the human being informs the direction that socialization will take. In this sense, socialization seeks to both construct and
reproduce that culture's ideal human being.

The consuming rational actor

What about our culture – the Western world at the beginning of the twenty-
first century? What is our dominant conception of the human being and
how is it constructed? There can be little doubt that there has never been
a society so subjected to normative and cajoling exhortations as ours. We
inhabit an almost all-pervasive media-penetrated conceptual and symbolic
social environment saturated with the demands and images of consumerism. Through radio, television, newspapers, magazines, internet, posters,
billboards, corporate logos on our clothes and our commodities, corporate
sponsorship of public events, sports kits, sports stars, celebrity endorsements
and on and on, it is fair to say that there has never been a human generation
so subjected to a single existential imperative – consumption.

Consumerism is enacted not just as a series of actions but has become
virtually a state of being. We *are* consumers in our very orientation to the
world, in our very conceptualizations of the good life and in what we think
constitutes happiness and security. Consumerism has colonized our private
and public rituals, our very dreams and longings. The lottery millionaire
has become the epitome of success, of sudden enlightenment, the embodi-
ment of what is possible for each of us. Consumption is constructed and
widely believed to be the road to well-being and to the fulfilled life. What
we consume and how we consume have become the identifiers and markers of our social success, of our individuality, of our true selves and of our
social status. In short, the purpose of life has become for most of us to
consume. Not to be able to consume by extension identifies the failed life,
even the failed human being. Choosing not to consume is the mark of the
drop-out, the deviant and the socially maladjusted.

Creating and maintaining consumerism as an existential state is required in order to maintain the Western economic system. This system is one based on continual economic growth.[3] Annual economic growth is needed in order to meet corporate and state debts, generate capital, maintain the debt-based money system and secure profits. Powerful institutions such as the media become the vehicles by which ever new consumer needs and wants are stimulated and brought into being. Consumers are obliged to live in a constant artificially induced tension to have more in order to be more. Marketing and public relations have become the wizard diviners and enchanters of this system of belief.

One consequence (indeed manifestation) of this all-encompassing system is the dominance in public discourse of a certain version of economic rationality. This rationality elevates the functioning of a theoretically imagined free market economy to be the epitome of sound social behaviour. Concepts such as competition, efficiency, free choice, privatisation and many others have been elevated to a non-problematic status as guarantors of our normatively declared pursuit of prolonged economic growth as the privileged provider of social well-being. The logic of the free-market is asserted to be the most rational logic available – anything else becomes, *ipso facto*, irrational and potentially dysfunctional. This claim has its roots in the old Adam Smith assumption that each individual pursuing his or her own maximum utility results in optimum social well-being for all. The State's role is merely to ensure the best environment within which this rationality can proceed.

What has happened is that the rules of a particular economic language game have overwhelmed our ability to speak politically in any other credible way. Those who attempt to do so can be charged with being unreasonable, unrealistic, and even dangerous. The effect on public discourse of this ascendancy has been to close down the capacity to speak credibly in any

---

3   No book has better and most straightforwardly described this than E. F. Schumacher's wonderful book *Small is Beautiful: A Study of Economics as if People Mattered* (1973), London: Abacus. For a more modern treatment of the same topic see, for example, Richard Douthwaite (1992), *The Growth Illusion*, Dublin: Lilliput Press.

other categories. Thus even previously non-commoditized public services such as health and education must now be judged and valued according to free market and consumerist criteria. Privatization, by which public services are delivered as though they were consumable commodities, is assumed unquestioningly to be the means by which the services will be best and most 'efficiently' delivered. After all, the market cannot be wrong. The result is that most public discussion and political debate has become caught in an intellectual box beyond which one cannot meaningfully manoeuvre.[4]

Our dysfunctional system

The extraordinary thing about all of this is that the economic growth system is demonstrably not working. This is clear not just when we take a global perspective but is even increasingly apparent for those living in the West itself. Modern industrial society is socially and ecologically unsustainable. Data on this is overwhelming and barely needs repeating. A few brief illustrations will suffice. For example, it is now widely acknowledged that human induced carbon dioxide releases have begun a rapid (in geological time) climate change sequence. The UN's Intergovernmental Panel on Climate Change accepts the possibility that average global temperatures may rise by almost six degrees centigrade by century's end. Despite many predictions and models, the fact is that we do not know where climate change will lead us. We do not know whether we are at the start of a runaway climate change event or whether, even if we wanted to, we can slow it

---

4   See my chapter further elaborating on this point: 'Civil society and political argument: how to make sense when no-one is listening', in Deiric O Broin and Peadar Kirby (eds) (2009), *Power, Dissent and Democracy – Civil Society and the State in Ireland*, Dublin: A. & A. Farmar Ltd. See also my chapter 'Problems in Achieving Dialogue: Cultural Misunderstandings in the Corrib Gas Dispute', in Ricca Edmondson and Henrike Rau (eds) (2008), *Environmental Argument and Cultural Difference – Locations, Fractures and Deliberations*, Bern: Peter Lang AG.

down. What we can anticipate is that this aggressive alteration of the earth's careful balance of natural systems will precipitate a climatic feedback that is inevitably going to reconfigure the benign environmental conditions that have given rise to the series of complex life-forms presently in existence, including ourselves.[5]

The planet's life-forms are in peril from other sources as well. The loss of natural ecosystems and habitats, together with the impact of a variety of pollution sources, has directly caused an extraordinary extinction of species. In 1992, the biologist Edward Wilson estimated that 27,000 species were being lost each year. But by the end of 2001, BBC 1's *State of the Planet* documentary warned that the situation was far worse. It asserted that unless radical corrective steps were now taken up to a half of all the species on the planet would be lost within the next fifty to 100 years. The extermination of a species is irreversible. In truth, we don't know how many species there are nor therefore can we definitively know just how many are being lost. What we do know is that the reduction of bio-diversity is now occurring on a scale greater than any experienced in the last 65 million years and is directly the consequence of human activity.

Not only does our dominant system produce environmental unsustainability it also gives rise to dramatic social unsustainability. The planet simply cannot provide for Western patterns of consumption to be applied everywhere. At the turn of the new century, the world's richest countries, with 20 per cent of global population, accounted for 86 per cent of private consumption. The poorest 20 per cent accounted for 1.3 per cent of private consumption (*UN State of the World Population Report 2001*). Nearly 60 per cent of people in poorer counties lacked basic sanitation (approximately 2.6 billion people). A third did not have access to clean water. It is doubtful whether food production can be increased to meet the needs of an expand-

5   For gloomy but credible analyses of this see James Lovelock (2006), *The Revenge of Gaia*, London: Penguin. See also James Lovelock (2009), *The Vanishing Face of Gaia – A Final Warning*, London: Allen Lane. For a moderate economic analysis of this see the *Stern Review on the Economics of Climate Change* (2006), London: HM Treasury.

ing global population given the context of topsoil depletion, loss of fresh water supplies and a rapid decline in the supply of cheap oil.

All of these figures and issues have been well presented elsewhere. They will be referred to again in Chapter Seven. The point is that the economic system within which we are embedded and which is in large part socializing us, is producing death and destruction on an incredible scale. In terms of the concerns which are the subject of this book, it is giving rise to a crisis of care and compassion on a planetary and social level. Our ability as human beings to relate compassionately to each other and to the natural world around us has become deeply impaired directly because of a dysfunctional and unsustainable system.

Yet as individuals we are at a moral and ethical level no worse or no better than any individual who has gone before us in any previous culture. The problem for us is that our difficulties are *structural and systemic* in character and our system, unlike any which has preceded us, is all-pervasive and incredibly powerful. The consequence is that the ideas we have regarding what the good life is and how human beings should live in order to attain that version of the good life can now be significantly pursued and implemented in the short-term with little acknowledgement of limit or constraint.

These dominant ideas of what constitutes humanity are rooted in an amalgam of sources. Among these are Cartesian dualism (with its division between a privileged consciousness and inert matter); the legacy of the mechanistic and reductionist science of Bacon and Newton; the anthropocentric conception of God in the Judeo-Christian tradition; the primacy of particular modes of rational-instrumental forms of knowing; the historical impact of the patriarchal assumption of the superiority of men. This broad paradigm has worked itself out within a raft of self-referential social sciences. The negative social and ecological consequences of this have been most apparent in modern economic theory which is predicated on a series of assumptions such as in its treatment of natural resources as non-cost income, and in classical political theory which has privileged the concept of Nation-State sovereignty. Equally, too, patriarchy has marginalized women and those attributes constructed as specific characteristics of women, such as care. For this reason, it is often women who bear the greater responsibility for the practice of care and, in similar fashion, care itself may be perceived as a marginal activity best confined to the domestic or interpersonal sphere.

The consequence is that, by becoming enclosed within ever expanding and apparently successful social systems, those with political and economic power no longer comprehend the fragility or limits of the wider natural and social settings within which we must operate. Their apprehension of the world has become phenomenologically suspect. Nowhere is this more apparent than, as noted above, in the concept of Gross Domestic Product as a measure of material well-being. This index limits itself to a recording of the value of traded goods and services within a territorially bounded economy but cannot record pollution, resource depletion, bio-diversity loss or even real levels of human well-being.

But if evidence of unsustainability and dysfunction is so apparent why do the electorates of the 'democratic' world not insist on change? The answer to this is undoubtedly complex. It must include the observation that not enough see the need partly because the Western economic and political system continues to give the appearance of being largely successful despite the recent financial crises. Furthermore, it is difficult for many to imagine what an alternative society might look like. There is a natural fear of change, especially of systemic change. On a practical level, the levers of change, the political mechanisms by which change on the scale required can be effected, are in the possession of powerful State and corporate interests who do not want any change whatsoever.

But one very powerful explanation is that we are in the grip of a narrow and demonstrably false conception of the human being as self-interested and perforce obliged to be and almost entitled to be, at least in terms of practical living, largely indifferent to the fate and well-being of others who are outside our network of social relations. This constructed conception furthermore posits care and compassion as laudable theoretically but impractical and effete if applied socio-politically or globally. Compassion cannot be policy because it is out of synch with how the world 'really is' and with 'human nature'. This world cannot be changed. It is as it is. Our only obligation is to survive in it and ensure at least our own personal and familial well-being. In this conception, altruism is a strategy that leads to failure not success.[6]

We have thus come to dwell in a world of fear, a fear which in turn accentuates these impulses to narrow self-protection and self-enhancement.

> The phenomenological manifestations of this crisis present an awesome specter: emptiness, loneliness, fear, anxiety, aggressiveness without objectives, in a word, general dissatisfaction. Emptiness is born of a feeling of impotence, that there is little we can do to change our own life and that of society, and finally, that nothing is important. Loneliness is expressive of the loss of contact with nature and others in terms of friendship and gentleness; there is the lack of courage to commit ourselves. Fear is the fruit of the objective threats to life, to employment, to the collective survival of humanity in general. Anxiety has its origin in imagined fear, ignorance as to what one ought to do, in whom to trust, and what to expect; when anxiety grips an entire society, it means that the whole society feels threatened and senses its approaching end. Generalised aggressiveness reveals a rupture with the norms of relationship without which a society cannot be built or defended; what results is anonymity and the loss of the meaning of the Self; that is the worth and sacredness of the human person. (Boff 1982: 5)

Part of the problem here may be that we have misread the meaning of Charles Darwin's theory of natural selection. More accurately, we have allowed a false understanding of his work to be constructed, one that emphasizes certain purported political implications which conveniently suit this dominant ideological paradigm. Thus, we are led to think that Darwinism sanctions selfishness, the survival of the fittest and inherent competiveness. But even if these evolutionary components of natural selection are applied to human beings (there is in fact as much evidence in favour of co-operation and reciprocity), the empirical reality is that we are not

---

6   Consider what the reaction would be if the US President chose to divert the majority of the US military budget into food development aid. It would not be considered rational behaviour by US policy makers and would never be 'politically' possible. This type of calculation at the macro policy level is replicated right down to the household budget level. We do not give up flying aeroplanes for holidays abroad even though we know it would improve the environment and allow us mobilize resources for private donations to aid development elsewhere.

bound by them. These refer to our *biological* evolution. As noted above, the truth is that human beings – the product indeed of natural selection – operate *socially and culturally* and accordingly can and do 're-code' their behaviour in the light of social norms. Our biology is socialized.

Image of the isolated human subject

For some centuries now, we in the West have been living out of a deeply limited conception of what it is to be human. The legacy of Descartes has left us believing that we are minds bound within bodies and that our unique private consciousness affords us a privileged perspective on the world. Nowhere is this Cartesian image of the isolated individual so wonderfully realized and depicted as in the mature work of Samuel Beckett. His magnificent post-war trilogy of novels – *Molloy*, *Malone Dies* and *The Unnameable* – are the profoundest meditations into the solitary Cartesian consciousness undertaken anywhere in modern Western culture. His deeply unsettling play *Endgame* similarly depicts isolated human beings clinging on to their remaining shreds of consciousness while the social and ecological world about them has fallen apart. Though the central character Hamm knows this, he is incapable of escaping from the prison and torments of his own mind and is unable to relate to other people other than as props and objects in the invented drama of his life. He is a lone chess player who has lost the game but must play out the final, inevitable moves (hence the title 'endgame'). Thus, he muses alone to himself, invents pointless rituals and dramas, torments his servant Clov and confines his hapless parents to two dustbins.

> Hamm: Can there be misery – [*he yawns*] – loftier than mine? No doubt. Formerly. But now? [*Pause.*] My father? [*Pause.*] My mother? [*Pause.*] My ... dog? [*Pause.*] Oh I am willing to believe they suffer as much as such creatures can suffer. But does that mean their sufferings equal mine? No doubt. [*Pause.*] No, all is a – [*he yawns*] – bsolute, [*proudly*] the bigger a man is the fuller he is. [*Pause. Gloomily.*] And the emptier.

The existential reality that results from (or is created by) this isolated consciousness is outlined by Hamm in a later speech when he prophesies the inevitable future for his downtrodden servant Clov:

> One day you'll be blind, like me. You'll be sitting there, a speck in the void, in the dark, for ever, like me. [*Pause.*] One day you'll say to yourself, I'm tired, I'll sit down, and you'll go and sit down. Then you'll say, I'm hungry, I'll get up and get something to eat. But you won't get up. You'll say, I shouldn't have sat down, but since I have I'll sit on a little longer, then I'll get up and get something to eat. But you won't get up and you won't get anything to eat. [*Pause.*] You'll look at the wall a while, then you'll say, I'll close my eyes, perhaps have a little sleep, after that I'll feel better, and you'll close them. And when you open them again there'll be no wall any more. [*Pause.*] Infinite emptiness will be all around you, all the resurrected dead of all the ages wouldn't fill it, and there you'll be like a little bit of grit in the middle of the steppe. [*Pause.*] Yes, one day you'll know what it is, you'll be like me, except that you won't have anyone with you, because you won't have had pity on anyone and because there won't be anyone left to have pity on.

These extraordinary lines provide a stark image of a Cartesian world of solitary conscious subjects who are devoid of empathy and compassion. In such a world, each of us lives in a defined geometric space, enclosed within our own consciousness, ultimately removed from each other. This is a world where care barely exists, overwhelmed by each individual's final inability to escape the constraints and obsessions of one's own mind.

Like all great artists Beckett both captures and evokes the world in which we live. Beckett's work shows us what this world looks like and feels like. In approaching Beckett's work we are both struck by the depth of his insights into our humanity and the grim humour to be derived from it but we are also repelled by the despair and the savagery of the human situations depicted. Yet, even in Beckett, there is always the possibility that this isolation and harshness is not all that can be said about us. There is also companionship, shared journeying, even the possibility that the Cartesian consciousness is wrong. Thus, Vladimir muses in *Waiting for Godot*:

> Was I sleeping, while the others suffered? Am I sleeping now? Tomorrow, when I wake, or think I do, what shall I say of today? That with Estragon my friend, at this place until the fall of night, I waited for Godot? That Pozzo passed, with his carrier, and that he spoke to us? Probably. But in all that what truth will there be?

In confronting the Cartesian conception of the human being and its socially constructed off-spring the rational, self-interested actor we can pose to ourselves this searing question of Vladimir's – 'But in all that what truth will there be?' Once again, as noted above, the essential issue is – do we have a correct conception of the human being? Can we transcend the limits of our ideological conditioning and gain a new perspective on ourselves?

Care as key constituent of humanity

To do so we need to start with an empirical rigour which would require us to pay close attention to the world as it actually is beneath the veneer of form and illusion. Can we, to deploy the language of Wittgenstein, clear up our confusions and truly see what lies open to view?

Perhaps, however, there is no privileged perspective and we must inevitably end up contesting and arguing about ourselves and our humanity. Yet even if this is so, I want to argue that care and compassion are fundamental human characteristics. Indeed, I think that care and compassion are so fundamental that they are constitutive of humanity itself. However, I think that this is more than just an assertion – it can be empirically demonstrated.

We can start with a simple thought experiment. Which world would you like to live in – one where everyone is cared for or one where there is no care whatever? When faced with an absolutely clear choice between a universe of care and one of indifference, which one would we be likely to choose? The Gulags and Auschwitz are our contemporary images of hell, places where terror and cruelty reigned and where little pity, mercy or compassion was found. Would anyone really choose to live in the world of the camps rather than in a liberal, tolerant, democratic society? While human beings have created all of this, and other human beings have suffered in all of this, we cannot doubt where we would better find humanization. We are capable of constructing both extremes but can we truly doubt which one better represents the beings we would like to be? The camps de-humanize both their creators and their victims. They are designed to de-humanize, to render persons into objects, into categories and into numbers.

Which would we naturally prefer – to be among people who are kind, considerate and truthful or those who are harsh, aggressive and vindictive? It seems to me apparent that, *when faced with the clear choice*, we are naturally pre-disposed towards those who are caring. We naturally prefer co-operation to conflict, peace to violence and agreement to dissension. These preferences are apparent as states that we strive for, as preferential conditions for our lived experience. They represent our default position, the condition of stability and security that we regard as our 'steady state' position. It is in this preferred condition that we can allow ourselves to eat without constant vigilance and to sleep without wakeful anxiety.

It seems to me that these observations are grounded in our existential reality and in any comprehensive phenomenological analysis of human society and behaviour. The evidence is there that human beings seek to create social worlds that are ordered and secure rather than chaotic and disturbed. That this is so is not a trivial observation. It necessarily points to something important about us. Though this may strike the reader as stating the obvious nevertheless, as the novelist and philosopher Iris Murdoch wisely noted, sometimes stating the obvious is important.

In similar vein we can develop our observations of the everyday world further and discover precisely in what way care and caring are intrinsic features of our humanity. For a start, no human child can survive biologically, or develop in a psychologically healthy manner, without care. Even allowing for the many and varied circumstances by which children are conceived, it is not unreasonable to assume that the great majority are conceived in acts of love. For the child to develop in the womb, the mother must be caring and nurturing of herself and of the new life within her. After birth, the child is entirely dependent on other human beings. It must be cared for otherwise, quite simply, it will not survive. It must be fed, kept warm, spoken to, held and protected from threats. Indifference is simply not a strategy for survival or human development. The fact of the matter is that without care there would be no human beings at all. That is the truth of it.[7]

The nurturing and caring of a child, whether done by mother, father, extended relatives or others, provide us with the primordial images and experiences of care. Responding to a cry; feeding; holding; tickling; playing; comforting; protecting; hushing; singing; all of these and more are the fundamental repertoire of care intrinsic to most human beings. The world after all is full of mothers and fathers. It is therefore full of people who have spent years fixed on attentiveness to a vulnerable other. And, of course, the world is full of people whose earliest experiences are of receiving care and comfort. Thus it can legitimately be said that (other than for certain limited exceptions the appalling effects of which are well known) each and every human being's primordial experience is one of *being cared for*. It can also legitimately be said (again with exceptions of course) that every father and mother's primary experience is one of *caring for*.

Thus the most fundamental human experiences are deeply grounded in care. Without early childhood care – love, acceptance, nurturing – there is something possibly irretrievably stunted in our human development. So much of our observed mental illness and distress almost certainly have their origins in early childhood experiences and predominantly are found among those who have been deprived of appropriate early care. These primal experiences of care through which our minds and bodies mature are perhaps so powerful that, even as adults, we are all yearning for the safety and security of simply being unconditionally cared for again. Perhaps it is this deep longing that lies at the heart of the almost universal phenomenon of religion and religious belief. Most cultures assert a belief system that suggests that the universe itself, despite all our sufferings and all the evil that we witness, is nevertheless somehow fundamentally characterized by care and concern.

---

7   See the Zeitgeist documentary film *Moving Forward* (2011) for an accessible treatment of the contemporary neuroscientific evidence regarding the necessity of care for healthy childhood development.

I do not want to push these observations too far. However, given the ubiquity and necessity of care in the development of human beings, it cannot be suggested that care is some add-on luxury or late evolved feature of human culture. On the contrary, it seems to me that *there cannot be any sociality without care*. Caring permits us to nurture our young, protect our old (who are our repositories of wisdom and tradition) and safeguard our weak and ill until they are well again. It is care that leads us to carefully and considerately attend to our dead and mourn their passing. We do not unthinkingly discard our corpses on the ground. Without this mutual commitment to care for others in order that others care for us, it is almost impossible to conceive how sociality in any complex manner could have developed. In addition, socially appropriate behaviours such as telling the truth, being trustworthy, not taking advantage of another's vulnerability, being generous, showing solidarity, working with others seem to me absolutely fundamental prerequisites for any cultural formation. Without these essential social connections we would indeed be plunged into the Hobbesian dystopia of everyone at war with everyone else in lives that were nasty, brutish and short. Yet, if this Hobbesian vision of our lives were true, we could barely have formed any social grouping in the first place. Our very sociality itself is strong evidence for mutuality and caring as constitutive of our humanity.

As noted in the Introduction above, we are powerfully predisposed to fit in with our social groups and wider culture. Our language, our accents, our dress codes, our etiquette, values, norms and even our dreams, are all socially given to us. We pay close attention, often quite unconsciously, to all of this complex mosaic of social rules and conventions so that we can be recognized as participants in the meaningful universe of our shared human society. We cannot be indifferent to this. We must care, contribute and cooperate with others in order to belong. Our sociality defines us, civilizes us and humanizes us.

At far more intimate levels we seek each other out for love and emotional connection. The thrilling realms of love, courtship and sexuality draw us inexorably towards each other and have allowed us to develop a complex repertoire of adult affection and playfulness. Being uncaring and self-centred within these realms is generally speaking a poor stratagem unlikely to be rewarded with fulfilling and stable relationships.

Most human beings have incredibly strong responses of compassion for the vulnerable and hurt. Crying, hunger, thirst, pain – these experiences in another person draw deep reactions from us. It is almost impossible for us to look into the eyes of someone hurt or frightened without some emotional response on our part. We are profoundly affected by the eyes and faces of others. Is it not that in them we can see ourselves too? The cries and calls for help of another person who is in immediate danger whether from drowning or falling provoke an almost automatic desire in us to assist.

David Grossman's fascinating study of men in war situations, *On Killing*,[8] finds that, contrary to popular assumptions, ordinary men actually find it virtually impossible to kill another man. Only 2–4 per cent can do so without suffering serious psychological damage. A key factor is whether they can see the eyes of the other. The more *distant* they are from their victim the easier it is to kill. For this reason, to be effective in combat soldiers have to be highly trained and conditioned. The purpose of this is to de-sensitize them to inflicting harm on another person and to overcome their instinctive empathic reactions to others.

We are in fact highly empathic beings, as we simply must be in order to form coherent, secure social groups and societies. The deep extent of our empathic structures can be seen even in the way we respond to fictional constructions of our own imagination. Just note the responses we have to characters and situations in novels, plays and films. We feel the fear and terror, we vicariously experience the love and heartbreak, to such an extent that we can jump with fright or cry real tears in response to fictional plots and dramas. All of this – the very capacity to create fiction and art in the first place – testifies to our deep inherent empathic responses. We can feel ourselves in the place of another person – feel their pain, their fear, their loss. Were we not to have these capacities we would be sociopathic,

---

8   David Grossman (1995), *On Killing: The Psychological Cost of Learning to Kill in War and Society*, Back Bay Books, Little, Brown and Company.

psychopathic and utterly unable, if these traits were found among many of us, to form any meaningful society at all.

Indeed we are so intrinsically empathic that we probably have to consciously ration or limit our compassionate responses otherwise we would be simply overwhelmed. This 'economy of love' by which we must select those to whom we relate in a caring manner is a more pronounced feature of modern societies because they are characterized by large aggregations of people within highly complex and stratified social relations. Thus we can pass a crying person on an urban street where we would be unlikely to do so if we encountered them on a solitary rural lane. Given the sheer numbers of us, we simply cannot care for everybody equally. We must choose.

The 'economy of love' concept is important as it may help to explain behaviour which otherwise seems cold and callous. It also may help to explain how we can rationalize our own behaviour to ourselves when we turn a blind eye to the palpable and visible sufferings of others about us. We say to ourselves 'there is so much need and I can only do so much. My first duty is to my own family and neighbours'. But what is crucial here to understand is that we behave in this more calculated manner not because we are at first instance uncaring and self-interested but, on the contrary, because we are so potentially full of empathy and compassion that we would be rendered incapacitated if we tried to respond to all claims of care upon us. We must deliberately shut down our receptivity to others and be selective in our responses otherwise we would be thoroughly overwhelmed with empathic demands which would make our own lives practically impossible to live.

We should not confuse however this pragmatic strategy with a principled refusal to care. The majority of people do indeed care at a personal level but calculate that modern society has in place specific institutions designed to respond to all citizens in need. In this sense at least, it is assumed that modern societies are designed to provide maximum social care and with this comfort and consolation in mind most citizens go about their own business and reconcile themselves to a necessary rationing of their own personal expressions of care.

For this reason, much of our practice of care which formerly was expressed within the interpersonal life-world of the individual, has now been transferred or delegated to various social institutions. There has been no diminution in our personal capacity to care. If there is a problem in care today it is a social one not a personal one.

The creation of dedicated institutions of care does not of course mean that when confronted with a specific instance of lack of care most citizens will not become outraged. Implicitly, we draw on a fundamental sense of what is right in our treatment of people. This innate moral disposition is also testimony to the powerful impulses of compassion embedded within us. These impulses come strongly to the fore when, for example, we are confronted with any natural or human-made disaster. Just consider how people immediately and spontaneously respond to crisis situations such as flooding, earthquakes and famines. There is a natural reflex to care and act and reach out to those in need. We have seen this in the south-east Asian tsunami, the Haitian, New Zealand and Japanese earthquakes and to flooding events which have occurred recently in parts of Europe and, of course, most dreadfully in Pakistan. The point is that people's default position is one of care and solidarity not self-interested protection. Disaster and communal crises return us to our deep human roots and we tend to respond accordingly. We don't have to be told to do this – it comes quite naturally.[9]

We can therefore understand why many important modern philosophers such as Martin Heidegger regarded care as fundamental dispositions of the human existing subject. It is our capacity to care that propels us forward in our own existence, directs us into projects that shape and determine our lives, and makes us concerned about the future. Heidegger argues that if we did not care we could barely exist in a meaningful sense. Without caring we would simply be in the world as though we were objects. We would be inert and passive. Our very subjectivity, our capacity to work on the world in which we find ourselves, is the product of our elementary disposition towards care. We have a fundamental concern with how things are about us. We shape the situations about us in order to render them

9   See Jeremy Rifkin (2009), *The Empathic Civilization*, Cambridge: Polity Press.

more in line with our desires and concerns. Without this commitment and engagement what kind of beings would we be?

Of course it is not just modern philosophy which offers us these insights. The great traditional religions of the world all place compassion and care at the heart of their religious practice. Whatever about their ultimate metaphysical truth or not, the great religions nonetheless capture and express fundamental insights into the nature of human existence. They encapsulate many centuries and millennia of reflection on the human condition. Irrespective of their doctrinal and dogmatic differences, all of them unite around certain core proposals that human fulfillment is achieved through a commitment to the well-being of others, through a letting go of self-interest and ego, and through a recognition that we are all bound up with each other as brothers and sisters. Indeed, it is remarkable the commonalities among the great religions on these themes. Once again, I believe that this is not a trivial observation and that something profound and significant is contained in these ideals which have remained potent and meaningful over some thousands of years.

In this way, the various world religions can be cited as further phenomenological evidence for the intrinsic nature of care. While the different religions may ground care and compassion as a response to the divine or to the ultimate nature of reality, the key insight to be gleaned for our purposes is how distinctive cultures in diverse social settings and historical periods nonetheless assert the practice of care and compassion as at the heart of humanization and religious enlightenment. That seems to me to be teaching deserving of the highest possible respect and not to be lightly dismissed.

Within the Christian tradition the incarnation of Jesus of Nazareth who, though God, became human in order to enter our experience, was poor, and died the death of an outcast prisoner serves for Christians as the supreme exemplification of care in action. Here is an extraordinary historical manifestation of God as a failure and a social reject. This is a God who seeks out the place of maximum public humiliation. There is a choice made here by him to identify fully with the poor and oppressed of history. God in the person of Jesus of Nazareth enters directly and fully into their specific experience.

The crucifixion is the central event in the Christian gospels. In confronting and accepting death by crucifixion it is clear that Jesus made a conscious decision not to evade this experience. He could after all have run away and lived for another day. He could have spoken out and tried to incite the crowds to protect him and confront his enemies. He could have resisted by organizing and arming his followers. He could have attempted to seek religious and political power. Instead he meekly submitted to his fate and died a similar death to that of millions of unknown poor people down through history.

The reason for this choice could only be because he chose to manifest God's extraordinary compassion, to show that God suffers exactly as we suffer. He chose to be present at the point of utter suffering and oppression and to thereby declare to history that this is the very place where God is to be found – broken, tortured and executed.

What kind of God is this? The subversive memory contained within the Christian tradition defeats all conventional and standard historical or anthropological conceptualizations of God. I wonder do Christians have any idea how radical and extraordinary this God of theirs is? In the gospel of Matthew, chapter 25, Christians are told explicitly that Jesus is to be found among the hungry, the thirsty, the refugees and 'non-nationals', the materially poor, the sick, the prisoners. This was a huge shock to his contemporaries who expressed amazement and incredulity. Jesus' reply as recorded in the gospel is clear: 'I tell you the truth, whatever you did not do for one of the least of these, you did not do for me.' I dare say that today's Christians might still be shocked if they really considered the implications of these words.

In this context it is little surprise that one of the most fruitful and progressive currents in modern Christianity has emerged from the southern, poor world. This current is often grouped under the generic category of liberation theology. The spirituality of liberation that emerges from this theological perspective is well summarized in Roger Haight's book on liberation theology in his description of the work of Segundo Galilea.[10]

---

10   Roger Haight (1985), *An Alternative Vision – An Interpretation of Liberation Theology*, Mahwah, NJ: Paulist Press.

First of all, he stresses that a conversion to Christ can take place only through a conversion to our neighbour and to a commitment to those who suffer oppression. A second intuition insists that there exists a profound relationship between 'salvation history' and the genuine liberation of the poor in Latin America so that 'to commit oneself to the latter is to work together with Christ the Redeemer and to enter into his saving work.' Third, liberating tasks must be seen as an anticipation and advancement of the kingdom of God, a kingdom which is marked by justice, equality, fraternity, and solidarity. The fourth basic intuition envisions liberating praxis, that is, the activity which transforms society on behalf of the oppressed, as one of the most important exercises of Christian charity, since Christian love has to be incarnated and made efficacious in reality. Lastly, he emphasises the value of poverty, which is not only a sharing in the plight of the poor but also a sharing in their struggle for justice, and which implies accepting persecution as a form of poverty and of true identification with Christ. (Haight 1985: 236, citing Hennelly referring to Segundo Galilea's *Espiritualidad de la Liberación*, 1973)

If the Christian tradition is recovering its essential injunction to care for one's neighbour not just interpersonally but also socially and politically, it may also be recognized that the Buddhist tradition, particularly the Mahayana 'school', has placed compassion at the heart of its existential practice over all of its two and a half thousand years. For Buddhism, compassion begins with the recognition that all sentient beings suffer and that the response to this is to try and bring such suffering to an end, not just for oneself but for all. One of the great and noble exemplars of this Buddhist insight today is the 14th Dalai Lama. His simple yet compelling teachings on compassion are not just the naïve ideas of a dedicated monk but are also grounded on his lived experience as an exile, whose country is unjustly and cruelly oppressed and who has seen the wanton murder of many close friends and associates.

Compassion can be roughly defined in terms of a state of mind that is non-violent, nonharming, and nonaggressive. It is a mental attitude based on the wish for others to be free of their suffering and is associated with a sense of commitment, responsibility, and respect towards others ... [G]enuine compassion is based on the rationale that all human beings have an innate desire to be happy and overcome suffering, just like myself. And, just like myself, they have the natural right to fulfill this fundamental aspiration. On the basis of the recognition of this equality and commonality, you develop a sense of affinity and closeness with others. With this as a foundation, you can feel compassion regardless of whether you view the other person as a friend or an enemy. It is based on the other's fundamental rights rather than your own mental projection. Upon this basis, then, you will generate love and compassion. That's genuine compassion. (Dalai Lama & Howard C. Cutler: 1999: 91–2).

Buddhism's belief in re-birth has given rise to the beautiful image that every human being, when you consider the many thousands and thousands of previous lives we each have lived, can be regarded as once having been our mother or our child. My present child may once have been my mother; my present parent may once have been my child. If we consider each human being as my mother or as my child then would we not be fully caring and compassionate to everyone?

Later in this book we will briefly consider the question whether we indeed require a spirituality of care in order to practise integral social care. For now, however, my concern is to demonstrate how care and compassion, as fundamental values and practices, have been embedded within our most profound and mythic ideas about ourselves as humans. Our conception of the best human being, the most achieved and enlightened human being, found within virtually all religious traditions on the planet, has centred on these specific attributes. Thus these attributes of care cannot be regarded as alien characteristics foreign to our humanity but, on the contrary, are our most intimate and desired conceptualizations of ourselves. Our recent adherence to images of our humanity as self-interested and concerned with maximizing personal utility (a perspective which as we have seen is a fundamental assumption underpinning conventional economics) can in fact be regarded as an aberration and unusual in historical and anthropological terms.

As has been argued above, it is crucially important that we have correct and true understandings of ourselves. Such understandings serve not only as descriptions but also construct the idealizations that we aspire to achieve. If we believe ourselves to be individualized self-interested consumers then that is precisely what we will be. We will continue to enact the drama of *Endgame* and bring into reality the nightmare of our own fears. We will regard the circumstances and sufferings of others as their own responsibility and of little or no relevance to us.

Yet, having said all that, it is not unreasonable at this point to take stock of all of these assertions about the extent to which care is indeed fundamental. One can legitimately argue that if care is so basic to us, why is the world as it is? Why is there so much suffering, so much poverty and so much inequality and exclusion? The evidence of human horror, cruelty and indifference is all around us. The answer to this lies I think in recognizing that our problems with care are now primarily *social and structural* and that in order to fully manifest and practise care we need to acknowledge that, in our type of societies, care must not just be an inter-personal phenomenon it must also be political and social. We remain, as we have always been, individuals who are combinations of good and bad characteristics. Yet, in general, human beings treat the person before them with respect and forbearance. Our callousness is reserved for those whose eyes we never see and never can see and never wish to see – those who lie outside our 'tribe' or 'class'.

Modern society compartmentalizes and stratifies social existence so that the worlds of the wealthy and capable rarely interact in a meaningful sense with the world of the poor and incapacitated. The poor are invisible, present but not seen. Their whispers and shadows and signs are all about us but we avert our eyes according to the rationale of the 'economy of love'.

For this reason, love and care today, for us inhabitants of the twenty-first-century globalized world, must be political. Responding to today's Jesus surrogates of the hungry, thirsty and poor, cannot just be confined to the interpersonal level because this can never be fully enough and never be fully effective. Interpersonal care is necessary but it is not sufficient. For care to be truly effective it must be political because the solutions to most of today's national and global sufferings and oppressions are structural in nature. As argued above, conceptualizing care as encompassing both the interpersonal and the political is what is called in this book integral social care, and it requires compassionate activism. Compassionate activism is an option and challenge to be taken up by every citizen. It is not something just for a cohort of professional social carers.

This contention is one of the central themes of this book and will be further explored below. Before concluding this chapter however, we need to briefly address two questions that can usefully summarize what has just been examined in the chapter and that can help to orient our further discussions in the chapters to come. First, what do we mean by care? Second, why should we care at all? Should we not after all just look after ourselves and let each person be responsible for their own well-being?

Definition of care

Trying to attain a comprehensive understanding of care, particularly of social care, is the ultimate purpose of this book. In the final chapter, an effort will be made to describe the specific characteristics of the compassionate activist. For now, however, we need to offer a preliminary explanation of what is meant by integral social care.

As noted above, the term 'to care' may have a patronizing ring to it. It seems to imply pity and charity. However, genuine care must not centre on pity. Instead, the core objective of what it is to care for someone is to be concerned with their liberation, by which is meant their personal and social transformation so that they can be who they truly are as persons and exercise a maximum of freedom and autonomy. The very essence of care is to liberate the person from all that binds them, from all that oppresses them and from all that curtails their freedom to be truly themselves.

Thus care is a developmental, liberating endeavour. It seeks out the freedom of the other. It is about letting the other be fully human, liberated from the psychological and sociological oppressions that limit their humanity. In short, then, to care for someone is about participating in their integral liberation – personal and social – so that they can become fully human.

This endeavour centres on entering into relationships with another person that are authentic in their manner and liberating in their intent. These are two characteristics of the utmost importance. Authenticity means that we who purport to care in these relationships are ourselves fully human and fully real, and that we are genuinely present and open to the other. Not to be authentic implies that we are performing a role or adopting a mask. This might mean that we are pretending to care. If this is so, then these relationships will not succeed. They will be exposed as false and will inevitably flounder. In this case, we would become a further element in the oppression of the other person and leave them even more harmed than before. That would be unforgiveable. We will have more to say regarding authenticity and being real in the next chapter.

That these relationships be liberating implies that we enter into them with an explicit concern to assist in freeing the other from their psychological and social burdens and not to make them further dependent, least of all on us the carers. This is a long and complex process and those who formally or explicitly offer recognized care form merely one contributor to this process. But we need to know what we are trying to achieve. We need to know the purpose and point of social care. We need a yardstick so that we can measure our effectiveness. The answer I believe is that the more the other person becomes free from all that constrains them, in other words the more they become human, then the more effective our care has been.

Exploring what precisely is meant by being human forms the substance of Parts Two and Three of this book. As we have indicated, it will be argued that humanization involves an interpersonal dimension and also a socio-political one. We need to be attentive to both. In summary however, it can be suggested that the notion of being fully human is closely tied to the concept of freedom – the freedom to be oneself and the freedom to exercise life choices in accordance with one's own desires and capabilities. In this sense of course, humanization and freedom are open-ended processes. There is no final plateau that we ultimately attain or no pre-defined model for what it is to be human. We are all embarked together on the journey of freedom. Freedom does not come with a prescribed blueprint. It is not attained according to a pre-determined plan. Rather, it is a process to be discovered. It is created and explored and incarnated in the very dynamics of life itself, both personal and political. It is always before us to be encountered.

Thus, integral social care occurs when we recognize the humanity in each other and when we help each other achieve our full humanity. Integral social care relationships are characterized by mutuality. They involve a reciprocal exchange whereby we humanize each other. The carer is humanized by caring, the cared-for is humanized in receiving care. At different times, depending on circumstances, these roles can easily be reversed. Mutual humanization – the accentuation of compassion, empathy, tolerance – is what binds us together in these relationships. That is why, in integral social care, there can be no place for attitudes or behaviour that are patronizing or superior, or for the labeling of someone as deficient or defective. If these do occur then they no longer permit the relationship to be characterized as caring. On the contrary, they add further to the structure and experience of oppression.

As we have said, professional social care practice occurs within a wide variety of formal and institutional settings. Social care in this narrower vocational sense involves intentional care by a professional carer of a service user who has presented with specific and defined personal and/or social needs. Care in this context requires certain professional skills and competencies. These will be explored in detail in Chapters Four and Five. However, even in these formal settings, care must still be characterized by relationships that are authentic and liberating. Otherwise, there is a danger that we will 'pathologize' professional social care relationships and assume that they have utterly distinct features from any other form of caring relationship. While some elements may be particular, depending on the circumstances of the individuals concerned, the essential characteristics of professional care relationships are no different from any other form of integral social care dynamic. The skills and values required – acceptance, dialogue, authenticity, respect – are those that we deploy in all our serious and meaningful relationships. Effective care is not the product of professionalization – it is the product of humanization.

However, it should be stated that entering into an intentional integral social care relationship with another person is an endeavour of the utmost gravity. Our capacity to do harm to another, however unwittingly, should never be underestimated. Entering into the life of another person, especially someone who may be vulnerable, is a delicate and serious enterprise. It should not be done lightly or without thought. Any work undertaken with other human beings is a moral activity involving a commitment to ethics, to appropriate interpersonal relations and to sound personal and political judgement.

Why should we care at all?

The argument of this chapter has been that care, rather than being an optional feature of human behaviour, to be undertaken only when all our basic needs are met, is in fact integral to, and constitutive of, our very humanity. From infancy on we survive only because of the care given to us by others. All of us attain our humanity because we are the recipients of care. We could not be who we are without care.

We should care for each other because that is who we are. If we close down care, diminish our caring instincts and render our societies places without care where indifference and isolation characterize our social relations, then we will diminish our own humanity.

Perhaps however there is no final way to intellectually prove this argument. If we do not intuitively grasp how intrinsic care is to us then no argument will suffice. In Albert Camus' great novel *The Plague* the Algerian city of Oran is depicted in the throes of a bubonic plague epidemic. The plague is a metaphor for totalitarian oppression but also serves as a metaphor for any form of social suffering. The townspeople are dying in huge numbers. What does one do in the face of this disaster? Does one care for those dying and suffering or does one seek only to save oneself?

The characters in the novel adopt different positions on this question. The Catholic priest Fr Paneloux interprets the plague as a divine punishment for human evil, something therefore we must simply accept as our just desserts. "'Calamity has come on you, my brethren, and my brethren, you have deserved it.'" Rambert, a young journalist, initially seeks only to abandon the city so that he can return to his own private happiness outside it. The disreputable character Cottard welcomes the plague because the collective catastrophe absolves him of personal responsibility to care for anyone – he is now equally condemned with everyone so why should he bother.

However, the most interesting character is the medical doctor Dr Bernard Rieux. He determines to resist the plague by directly caring for its victims. He organizes and co-ordinates 'sanitation squads' to help bring comfort and support to the plague victims. In the novel Rieux delivers some of the greatest but most sober lines of twentieth-century literature in support of human solidarity and compassion. While Rieux is described as 'fighting against creation as he found it' he himself only claims that 'The thing was to do your job as it should be done.'

> There are sick people and they need curing. Later on, perhaps, they'll think things over, and so shall I. But what's wanted now is to make them well. I defend them as best I can, that's all.

Opting out, being indifferent to the fate of others and ensuring his own personal welfare is not something considered by Rieux. His duty to others is clear. It does not require reasons or proofs. His lines finally explaining his position might perhaps serve as a modest statement of why one ought to care.

> There's no question of heroism in all this. It's a matter of common decency. That's an idea which may make some people smile, but the only means of fighting a plague is – common decency.

It is simply common decency to care. We all, I believe, know this. The complex nature of modernity and the necessity to develop an 'economy of love' can reduce and degrade our basic empathic and compassionate responses. That is something we need to become aware of which is precisely why we must recognize that integral social care operates not only interpersonally (which necessarily limits our caring opportunities) but also politically (which as citizens is the responsibility of all of us).

The extraordinary thing is that our myth fantasy about ourselves as self-reliant autonomous agents has blinded us to the truth that it is actually in our own self-interest to live in societies characterized by care and compassion. We all benefit. The humanity of each of us is enhanced by living in societies distinguished by harmony rather than by antagonism. This point will be further developed and detailed in Chapter Seven.

The truth is that we cannot just save ourselves. Human life is contingent, fragile, vulnerable and co-dependent. We each need support personally and socially. If not today, then tomorrow, it is we ourselves who may require to be cared for. As Thomas Merton reminds us, taking up John Donne's famous line 'no man is an island', without a culture and civilization of care we are all doomed:

> Never has the total solidarity of all men, either in good or in evil, been so obvious and so unavoidable. I believe we live in a time in which one cannot help making decisions for or against man, for or against life, for or against justice, for or against truth. (Thomas Merton, in acceptance of the Pax Medal 1963)

We are facing a crisis. It is systemic in nature encompassing politics, economics, ecology and our social world. In facing it, it is clear that we are not thinking deeply enough. We are guilty of 'fast thought'. The challenge before us is not simply re-tweaking or reforming some broken parts. Our system, and its various components, needs fundamental re-design.

The key concern in shaping this re-design is to determine exactly what we want our integrated social, economic and political system to do. We are no longer clear about this. This is one of the reasons why, despite the present system being clearly dysfunctional, we seem to be committed to somehow maintaining it despite all the evidence that it is not working. We are no longer seeing it correctly. Even if it could be sustained indefinitely, it should not. It is producing harm.

There are surely two key design objectives that we would want any system to achieve:

1. Social equality
2. Ecological well-being

Why are these critical? Because not only are they ethically appealing and appropriate, they are actually in each individual's ultimate self-interest. As we shall see below, social equality produces the best social outcomes across a range of issues and indicators and gives rise to the most human and secure societies. Ecological well-being is simply a fundamental prerequisite for life and happiness.

Our present system is producing antagonisms both within societies, between countries and between humanity and our planet. We need a system that produces harmonies. This is our challenge – to re-design our system to enhance harmony. Achieving harmony – social and ecological – is the political cause for today. That is the cause to which compassionate activists need to commit themselves. Compassionate activism is indeed a way to recover the nobility and utopian value of politics and to recover the belief that politics can be an instrument for positive social transformation.

We forget at our peril the utter simplicity of realizing that caring and being cared for are at the core of our humanity. They are the constituents of our well-being, the gateway to our own humanization. The complexity and stratification of modernity have misled us into a false image of ourselves and a curtailment of our natural empathy and compassion.

We now need to address in greater detail the critical questions previewed in this chapter: what precisely is it to care, and how do we do it?

PART TWO

The Interpersonal Dimension

CHAPTER THREE

Carl Rogers: A Framework for Personal Liberation

Within the broad disciplines of psychology and psychotherapy there are many methods and schools of thought. In this chapter, I propose to examine the concepts and means adopted by the American psychotherapist Carl Rogers.[1] I do so not necessarily because Rogers is obviously the best or most learned of psychological theorists but rather because his work, drawn from his decades of direct experience in writing, teaching and providing therapy, offers a rich and compelling account of what it is to become 'a person'. By 'person' Rogers means somebody who has truly become who they are and who therefore makes choices and communicates in a manner that is true to their sense of self. But Rogers' conceives of this 'becoming who you are' as an open-ended process of development and discovery. In a sense, his work is as much philosophical as it is psychological and has had a profound impact on modern social care both in its theory and in its practice.

It can reasonably be suggested that Rogers' key concern is with what constitutes a human being. As I have argued in the previous chapter, this is a question of the utmost importance in the context of integral social care. In order to be genuine and effective in our care, we clearly need to have a rigorous understanding of how we think human beings should be. We need to know this so that we can identify when dehumanization is apparent and in what general direction we regard humanization to lie. In other words, we need to have some criteria of distinction between what is more human and what is less human so that we properly and effectively orientate our practice of care. There is no question here of a blue-print of some kind, or

[1] Rogers was born in 1902 and died in 1987. He practised professionally from the 1920s, wrote many books and lectured in a number of US universities.

a template, or of some crude Procrustean standard. Rather, we necessarily require a coherent yardstick of judgement in regards to humanization and dehumanization. If we had no such criteria, even at an intuitive level, then we would merely be observers of our own collective and individual condition without imparting any values to that condition. That of course is not how we are or how we should be.

It is precisely in addressing these concerns that the value of Rogers' work can be found. Rogers is alert to the reality that humanization is best described as a process of becoming and that that process unfolds primarily within the dynamic of interpersonal relations. There is no fixed and final state of being that we must attain nor is the process of humanization a solitary, isolated task to be undertaken by an atomized individual. Instead, drawing on his professional experiences, Rogers identifies the general orientation along which humanization, conceived as an open process embedded within interpersonal relations, can be found. Of course, he is not the only psychologist to offer these or similar insights but the advantage with Rogers for our purposes is that his framework of understanding is sufficiently broad and inclusive to permit reflection and engagement with other, distinct perspectives.

The generating question driving Rogers' approach is how the human being becomes a person.[2] The theoretical framework within which he addresses this question is a broad humanistic one. In particular, Rogers draws from existentialist, phenomenological and person-centred approaches. Thus, based on these approaches, it is proposed that the person realizes his/her authentic identity by exercising his/her own free choices.

> [I]t appears that the goal the individual most wishes to achieve, the end which he knowingly and unknowingly pursues, is to become himself. (Rogers 1989: 108)

---

2   For the purposes of this chapter, we shall rely on Rogers' 1967 book *On Becoming a Person: A therapist's view of psychotherapy*. All references cited in this chapter are drawn from the 1989 edition of this text. Note that throughout Rogers uses gendered terminology when referring to human beings.

'Becoming himself' may strike the reader as having a somewhat trite and facile ring to it. However, Rogers argues that a shared characteristic of the people that he worked with in therapy was their tendency to adopt and hide behind false fronts, masks or roles. In order to be socially and personally acceptable – perhaps even to themselves also – they constructed a false view of themselves which became manifested in various personal practices and bahaviours. Illness and personal difficulties arose for such people due to the contradiction between these assumed behaviours and how they really wanted to be. Such people may not even have been aware that they were doing this nor may they necessarily have been consciously aware of who their true selves were. Thus, Rogers' person-centred approach is about working with the individual in order that they recover, or discover, who they themselves really are.

> He discovers that he exists only in response to the demands of others, that he seems to have no self of his own, that he is only trying to think, and feel, and behave in the way that others believe he ought to think, and feel and behave. (110)

The existential and psychological condition described here may be in fact quite common, one that we are all susceptible to at some level. As was noted in the Introduction above, we all exist in a tension between seeking to belong and seeking to be ourselves. For some, the yearning to belong – to fit in, to be acceptable – may completely overwhelm their sense of themselves. This may particularly happen where the individual is subjected to specific oppression by someone who has authority or power over them – a parent, a partner, companions, a boss, a bully. These figures of power may overtly insist that one ought to behave in a particular way, dress in a particular way, speak in a particular way, present themselves in a certain way, hold certain opinions, and so on. The inventory of possible oppressions is almost infinite. It may include various overtly conveyed social norms and expectations such as in regards to physical and intellectual ability, cultural homogeneity or sexual orientation. This insistence on adherence to someone else's standards effectively robs the individual of their own person. Hence, 'becoming himself' is far from trite and facile – it is the goal and task of all authentic human liberation.

Non-judgemental acceptance

The critical concept developed by Rogers of non-judgemental acceptance is not simply a therapeutic technique. It is rather the necessary condition that permits us to become a person. If we can accept each other as we are then we do not have to construct false fronts or masks of any kind. We can gift personhood to each other by simply accepting each other as we are and stopping our overwhelming tendency to judge, evaluate, improve and 'reform' each other.

> It is an atmosphere which simply demonstrates 'I care': not 'I care for you *if* you behave thus and so'. Standal has termed this attitude 'unconditional positive regard', since it has no conditions of worth attached to it ... it involves as much feeling of acceptance for the client's expression of negative, 'bad', painful, fearful, and abnormal feelings as for his expression of 'good', positive, mature, confidant and social feelings. It involves an acceptance of and a caring for the client as a *separate* person, with permission for him to have his own feelings and experiences, and to find his own meanings in them. (283)

Acceptance then becomes the key to personal growth and development because it gives the person permission to be themselves. They are accepted as a person without having to have recourse to false masks. This is incredibly liberating.

However, it is also incredibly difficult. To suspend all judgement when engaging with another person is immensely challenging. Each of us has almost an automatic reflex to evaluate, assess and categorize other people. Are they good or bad, threatening or safe, intelligent or foolish? These types of questions come spontaneously to our minds when dealing with others and, once again, they are an inherent aspect of our sociality.

True acceptance therefore requires attention and conscious decision. To achieve it we must lay aside our evaluative, judgemental responses and genuinely try to engage with the other person exactly as they are. This means to attempt to enter the other person's frames of reference in order to try and see from their perspective. This too is extraordinarily difficult but the effort must be made. It must be made because if we do not try and perceive as the other person perceives then we can never truly 'meet' them or truly encounter them. We cannot enter their subjectivity. We leave them before us as objects to be assessed and worked upon.

In truth, it is impossible of course to see fully through the eyes of another. But with dedication and empathy we can get close. The incredible difficulty of this endeavour should not be used as an excuse for not attempting it. After all, what is the alternative? If we proceed on the basis of 'judgemental acceptance' where will that leave us? It implies that we position ourselves over and above the other person and claim to be in a position to assess their lives and choices. It implies that we will accept them only on the basis that they fulfill certain conditions determined by us or by 'society'. Does this seem like a helpful, workable model for engaging with people?

Rogers is quite critical of a professionalization of care which seems to grant social permission for such judgement to occur and which has the additional consequence of positioning the carer at a distance from the person they are caring for. This professionalization seems to be based on a notion that too much empathy is potentially dangerous.

> Can I let myself experience positive attitudes toward this other person – attitudes of warmth, caring, liking, interest, respect? It is not easy. I find in myself, and feel that I see in others, a certain amount of fear of these feelings. We are afraid that if we let ourselves freely experience these positive feelings toward another we may be trapped by them. They may lead to demands on us or we may be disappointed in our trust, and these outcomes we fear. So as a reaction we tend to build up distance between ourselves and others – aloofness, a 'professional' attitude, an impersonal relationship.
>
> I feel quite strongly that one of the important reasons for the professionalization of every field is that it helps to keep this distance. In the clinical areas we develop elaborate diagnostic formulations, seeing the person as an object. In teaching and administration we develop all kinds of evaluative procedures, so that again the person is perceived as an object. In these ways, I believe, we can keep ourselves from experiencing the caring which would exist if we recognized the relationship as one between two persons. It is a real achievement when we can learn, even in certain relationships or at certain times in those relationships, that it is safe to care, that it is safe to relate to the other as a person for whom we have positive feelings. (52)

I think these are lines of great wisdom and insight. One of the most critical concerns in integral social care is that we ensure that we are agents of liberation for the other person and not agents of normalizing oppression. We must take stock and recognize that, in our actions, attitudes and omissions, we can serve one or other of these processes – liberation or oppression. We should not use our professional status as a distancing device absolving us of our fundamental duty to be participants in the liberation of the other person. There is no neutrality in this matter. If integral social care is centred on the objective of human liberation then its practices and processes must be liberating too.

However, we must be careful not to permit the concept of non-judgemental acceptance fall into caricature. Non-judgemental acceptance is not a blank cheque for bad behaviour. People do bad things and these should not be accepted. Other people can treat us too as objects and this should not be accepted. This, after all, dehumanizes us which defeats the interpersonal mutuality of integral care. As we have said, to dehumanize another is to dehumanize oneself and that applies to both care giver and care receiver. But the point is to carefully distinguish the person from their behaviour. Challenging behaviour is telling us something about the person. It is a form of communication and is almost always wrapped up in a fundamental defensiveness and inner fear or, if politically or socially motivated (e.g. prejudice), in ideological conditioning. Rogers is clear in his view that all people have a basically positive orientation and that the more they are accepted as persons 'the more he tends to drop the false fronts with which he has been meeting life, and the more he tends to move in a direction which is forward' (27).

This assertion can seem very difficult to accept especially for those who have been victims of cruel and destructive behaviour. It may also be very difficult to appreciate for those who must care domestically for a person who is totally incapacitated and behaving very cruelly to their carers. Yet it is only when you try and closely relate to even the most apparently heartless individual that you can nonetheless recognize the amount of humanity and care still present. Indeed, we may discover that much of the challenging behaviour manifested may well be a false front erected and internalized over many years in order to protect the person and insulate them from rejection and vulnerability. Nonetheless, relating to such individuals presents a troubling and difficult challenge because it may involve us having to overcome our natural emotional reactions to being ill-treated or exploited. That is why it is often an easier response to categorize certain people as 'all-bad' and as beyond redemption. But, other than in very limited and extreme cases, this is simply not true. After all, we have argued above that care is the fundamental grounding experience and preferential orientation for the great majority of human beings. For those few who have been so deprived of care as to render them now virtually sociopathic surely the appropriate response is not to further place them in care-deprived settings but to attempt to begin, with all its incredible and unsettling challenges, to reconstitute their fundamental human orientation towards care and compassion.

These are not easy ideas. Paradoxically, the setting and security provided by non-judgemental acceptance offers the very prerequisite that permits one to authentically and effectively confront the challenging behaviour of the other person. If you have conveyed that you have genuinely accepted the other person, that they are safe to be themselves with you, then, in that secure context, you are much more capable of critiquing challenging behaviours and thereby, within the dynamic of a caring authentic relationship, facilitating transformation. But if you *start* with criticism and judgement there is virtually no hope of effecting any transformation. If the latter was true, then we could 'solve' all personal problems by sitting people down and telling them their errors. We know that that simply does not work.

This discussion alerts us to a very important point. Caring and compassion are not easy. They are not for the faint-hearted. This is not a wishy-washy project for naïve 'do-gooders'. Care relationships are sometimes messy and complex and require toughness and commitment. After all, we may well be dealing with people who are angry, damaged, resentful and who forcibly resist any interactions and relationships. That is one of the reasons why I choose to use the term compassionate activism to designate integral social care, whether professional or otherwise. This term captures the type of determination and resilience required to enter into authentic caring relationships. To paraphrase the Christian gospel – if we only care for those who are 'nice' and 'deserving' what good is that. Anyone can do that. The real challenge is to care for those who are difficult and 'ugly'.

It is comforting of course if we can simply dismiss the difficult as unworthy of care. This might absolve us of any responsibility to them. This is a subtle and at times appealing temptation. After all, it is quite under-standable to recoil from hopelessness or rejection or aggression. At the end of the day it is not unreasonable to conclude that there is only so much one can do. While this line of reasoning is explicable, it may also be con-venient. While we cannot control the outcome or product of our integral social care relationships we can ensure, as long as they exist, that we remain committed to an authentic and liberating *process* of engagement. This is a point that will be developed in greater detail in the next chapter.

Much of this recoiling from the difficulties inherent in some care rela-tionships may have to do with fear on our part. I do not just mean physical fear. A more complex and often unacknowledged fear may be, as Rogers suggests, that our relationship with, and acceptance of, the other person may oblige us to change ourselves. Entering into authentic caring relationships, especially with the poor and oppressed, (in the sense in which these terms are used in this book) may require us to change our ideas, our attitudes, our sense of being right, sometimes perhaps our own social status. This may be deeply unsettling. It is for this reason that it is easier to discount them as hopeless and beyond any possibility of positive transformation.

Therefore, we need to be very self-aware and cautious if we are practis-ing care and compassion, to ensure that we do not regard it as something which is divisible and capable of being compartmentalized in this way. We either are committed to care for human beings or we are not. Sometimes we have a positive role to play in the humanizing of another and sometimes we do not. But we should not set up categories of the deserving and the non-deserving. It may well be that there are those who do not respond positively to a caring relationship or who consciously reject care. But, if we set limits *in advance* based on a pre-judgement rather than on experience and effort, then we are saying something clear about how committed to care we really are.

There are, in any event, natural constraints in place which regulates and restricts our care practice. For the professional care worker there are the boundaries set by his/her domain of work. The childcare worker works with children, the drugs councilor with addicts, and so forth. For all of us, whether professional or non-professional, the 'economy of love' within the interpersonal dimension places a natural limit on who, and how many people, we can directly relate to. There are only so many people we encounter and only so many that we can significantly respond to. But it is as citizens, in the socio-political dimension, that we can commit ourselves to ensuring that all are cared for without distinction. It is primarily in this dimension that we define how genuine is our commitment to integral social care. In this sense, non-judgemental acceptance is not just a personal norm and mode of relating to another person. It can also be conceived of as an appropriate social norm. As a society, as a political system, do we truly accept everyone as they are or might there be overt and covert discriminations and assumptions regarding 'normality' and acceptable identity built into our social policies and our laws? How are our sick, our 'disabled', our imprisoned, our refugees, our out of work, our nomads, actually treated? Are they accepted as they are? Are they treated in reality as human beings equal in dignity to every other citizen?

These reflections will be further considered below. One final point needs to be noted however. Non-judgemental acceptance as a principle and methodology refers not just to the other person, it also refers to ourselves. Do we truly accept ourselves exactly as we are? Or are we also forever constructing false fronts and masks in order to gain the acceptance of others? At issue here is our own humanization and our own process of becoming a person. We too are in issue in an authentic and liberating relationship. There is little value in us seeking to participate in the humanization of others if we ourselves are caught in an oppressed version of ourselves. We too must be who we authentically are.

> [T]he curious paradox is that when I accept myself as I am, then I change. I believe that I have learned this from my clients as well as within my own experience – that we cannot change, we cannot move away from what we are, until we thoroughly *accept* what we are. Then change seems to come about almost unnoticed.
>
> Another result which seems to grow out of being myself is that relationships then become real. Real relationships have an exciting way of being vital and meaningful ... Real relationships tend to change rather than to remain static. (17–18)

But how do we do this? How do we achieve this degree of personal liberation? There should be no doubt that, while this might be easy to put on paper and aspire to, it is incredibly difficult in practice. Also it should be clear that, given that we are dealing with *personal* liberation, it varies from individual to individual. Let us consider therefore Rogers' approach to realizing the authentic personality.

Emergence of the personality

As suggested above, there is no blueprint or template for the attainment of the authentic human person. Each individual is distinct and unique. Each individual is the product of their own personal circumstances and socio-political constraints and conditioning. Rogers' account therefore is one that outlines general characteristics or orientations. They are necessarily generalizations but are nonetheless drawn and validated from his direct experience over many decades.

Critically for Rogers, the process of becoming a person involves the individual in dropping the masks behind which they hide. The individual first must become aware of these masks and then slowly let them go in favour of their own authentic identity. This permits them to achieve the freedom to be themselves. Crucial to this process is that the person finds that as they dispense with false masks they are accepted as they really are. Through the liberating dynamic of non-judgemental relationships it is rendered safe and secure for them to be themselves. A key component in the unfolding of this process is that they must experience what they are actually feeling. This amounts to a 'discovery of unknown elements of self' (111). The person who then emerges can be described according to four general characteristics.

Openness to experience

Being open to experience refers, according to Rogers, to allowing oneself to become aware of feelings and attitudes as they arise and to an awareness of reality as it exists outside of oneself. Again, this may seem trite and somewhat obvious but when you consider it, it is in fact quite striking how people can be alienated from their own feelings and the world about them. What happens is that they filter or re-frame their feelings in order to make them acceptable or compatible to a pattern that they have decided upon or one that has been imposed upon them. Our tendency to judge and to evaluate come into play again and we fix our own selves and the world about us in accordance with preconceived categories.

> He is able to take in the evidence in a new situation, *as it is*, rather than distorting it to fit a pattern which he already holds. As you might expect, this increasing ability to be open to experience makes him far more realistic in dealing with new people, new situations, new problems. (115)

To genuinely be open to experience means being really engaged in what is actually going on about us without a predetermined interpretation. We often distort our perceptions of reality – 'I am happy', 'I do love that person', 'I am comfortable in this situation', 'There is nothing I can do about this', 'I agree with him' – because it is easy or causes less conflict. To truly be aware of what we are actually experiencing – whether it be anger, boredom, discomfort, fear – is potentially frightening because it may oblige us, and make us responsible, to bring about change. Deciding to avoid conflict and to fail to take responsibility are the major reasons why personal and political myths can take hold and be sustained. It is easier to filter out the dissonant and negative aspects of reality and remain enclosed in a comfortable state of delusion.

Thus people, though living in appalling circumstances, can often reconcile themselves to their situations. They may no longer even know what they are actually experiencing. Fear, powerlessness and oppression can easily be normalized. To quote Beckett again – 'habit is a great deadener'.

True openness to experience, without preconception or evaluation, is extremely difficult to both attain and sustain. It is almost a Zen-like state where one becomes completely present in the moment and thoroughly inside the experience of now. Our Western minds, with their endless chatter, distractions and projects, find this extremely difficult to achieve. Yet, Rogers is clear that 'this openness of awareness to what exists at *this moment* in *oneself* and in *the situation*' is a core characteristic of the emerging mature personality.

There can be little doubt that our feelings connect us to reality. Reality should not be thought of as a collection of objects before us. Rather, reality is something that we are always *relating to*. Our feelings are measures of the quality of that relating. If we suppress them, or organize them to make them compatible with our personal wishes or with wider social expectations, then we are losing important information about ourselves and the social setting that we are in. Our real, lived experiences tell us what is actually going on. Living in reality is always better than living in illusion and that is the ultimate condition for authenticity.[3]

Trust in one's organism

This observation leads Rogers to the second characteristic of the emerging person. Trusting in one's organism means trusting one's feelings, thoughts and body to accurately tell you what is happening. One can rely on this integral organic feedback to determine what decisions one should take. Only our own total organism can indicate to us who we are, what makes

---

3   Iris Murdoch showed in her philosophical work the enduring value of Plato's famous
    metaphor of the cave which describes the journey from illusion to truth as a move-
    ment away from the narrow egotistical concern with personal self-interest. In this
    rich metaphor truth and morality are seen to be correlated. In other words, the more
    one connects with reality the more virtuous one is. Self-absorption leads one into a
    state of delusion.

us the human being that we want to be and what it is that we are actually experiencing. Thus, if we are deeply unhappy in our present situation whether it is in a relationship, a career or a lifestyle we need to pay attention to our feelings and to our body. Unhappiness and illness may tell us that the life we are living is not one that really reflects the person we would like to be. But if we are closed to our own organism how can we possibly know who we are?

> To the extent that this person is open to all of his experience, he has access to all of the available data in the situation, on which to base his behavior. (118)

Of course our organism is not infallible and may get it wrong but 'because he tends to be open to his experiences, there is a greater and more immediate awareness of unsatisfying consequences, a quicker correction of choices which are in error' (118–19).

Having the confidence to trust in one's own organism and permitting others to trust in theirs suggests also an appropriate methodology for professional integral social care. The temptation for the social care professional to deploy and assert 'expertise', to impose solutions, to seek to 'fix' people based on a claim of privileged knowledge is almost always not the correct approach at all. Most people's own organism contains all the knowledge and insight that is required. Therefore, the task of the social carer is to free the person through non-judgemental acceptance to become the author of their own solutions and to encourage them to trust their personal organic experiences.

An internal locus of evaluation

This idea is closely linked to the claim that the emerging person should be their own evaluator. They should not seek approval or disapproval from others or from whether they conform to predetermined external standards. The source or location of their choices and decisions should be themselves.

He recognizes that it rests within himself to choose; that the only question which matters is, 'Am I living in a way which is deeply satisfying to me, and which truly expresses me?' This I think is perhaps *the* most important question for the creative individual. (119)

We can readily recognize in ourselves and in others this natural tendency to rely on others to evaluate decisions for us. Sometimes this involves following the crowd – doing what is the 'normal' (i.e. average) thing to do. Standing outside the crowd is extremely difficult. Again, if we go along with social expectations and judgements rather than our own we may well avoid conflict but the price to be paid is that we are not living from our own sense of ourselves. But why live a life other than your own?

There is great comfort and exhilaration in being a unique person, responsible for oneself. 'To recognize that "I am the one who chooses" and "I am the one who determines the value of an experience for me" is both an invigorating and a frightening realization' (122). In the post-war world it was Sartre who best recognized the extent to which human beings fear freedom because they fear the responsibility to choose which follows. We can often find greater comfort in being told what to do.

However, the authentic person must embrace his/her own freedom and escape from the evaluations of others. In a similar way, the compassionate activist must value human liberation and seek to always transcend the conditioning of our ideologically grounded social system. This theme is one that is further explored in Part Three of this book.

Willingness to be in a process

Finally, the emergence of the mature human person is a process. It is open-ended and never completed. The person is not a product who is made once and for all. They are a process, always becoming and always mysterious. Thus, we must never reduce any human person to a category. We must never consider that the last word has been spoken about them and that there is no more to be expected from them. Nothing is fixed and unalterable, least of all a person, even the very worst of people. Rather than narrowing people down to what they have been we should recognize that transformation and liberation is always a possibility on the wide horizon of each human existence.

> It means that a person is a fluid process, not a fixed and static entity; a flowing river of change, not a block of solid material; a continually changing constellation of potentialities, not a fixed quantity of traits. (122)

If we take these four general characteristics together, I believe we have an open, inclusive description of the human person. We have at least a working framework which allows us to determine the direction by which the process of humanization and dehumanization unfolds. At the minimum we can say that, in order for humanization to be underway, the person must be free in themselves to make their own choices, they should be accepted as they are, they should be free to follow their own course and they should be free of unreasonable external constraint.

Rogers' framework thus gives us a model for human liberation on the interpersonal level. It offers one possible but helpful yardstick by which we can measure the effectiveness of integral social care. If this is the case then we can say that integral social care is effective insofar as it facilitates the person to develop these four characteristics. If on the other hand it closes the person down, subjects them to external constraints, turns them into a product rather than accepting them as a process, renders them into an object rather than engages with them as a subject, then it is not bringing about human liberation but human oppression.

Congruence

The liberated person is, in Rogers' terms, congruent. The congruent person is one who can match or align their experience to both their awareness and to their communication with others. In short, they are aware of what they are experiencing and can communicate authentically from that awareness. The congruent person's 'I am', 'I know', 'I feel' ring true because it is spoken from their own direct encounter with themselves and the world. Thus, their communication with another is more likely to be clear and understood. There is less ambiguity from a congruent person. Such a person is best able to enter into open dialogue with another.

For Rogers, the greater the degree of congruence the person has the better their interpersonal relations will be. This principle he formulates into a general law as follows:

> The greater the congruence of experience, awareness and communication on the part of one individual, the more the ensuing relationship will involve: a tendency toward reciprocal communication with a quality of increasing congruence; a tendency toward more mutually accurate understanding of the communications; improved psychological adjustment and functioning in both parties; mutual satisfaction in the relationship.
>
> Conversely the greater the communicated *incongruence* of experience and awareness, the more the ensuing relationship will involve: further communication with the same quality; disintegration of accurate understanding, less adequate psychological adjustment and functioning in both parties; and mutual dissatisfaction in the relationship. (344–5)

Being congruent then regarding experience, awareness and communication is a necessary pre-condition for becoming oneself, for entering into authentic non-judgmental relationships and for facilitating the other person to in turn become themselves. Our being real helps others be real also.

In this modest sense at least we are responsible for our own liberation and, more significantly, we are each responsible for each other's. Rogers' emphasis here is on the *interpersonal* nature of becoming a person. Becoming a person is not, and cannot be, a solitary project for the isolated individual. We shape and affect each other by the extent to which we accept each other, or judge and evaluate each other. We therefore have it in our capacity, at the interpersonal level no less than the political level, to humanize or dehumanize each other. The compassionate activist is one who is committed to the cause of humanization. That commitment begins with themselves, through personal acceptance and congruence, and continues within the various interpersonal relationships that they are involved in and extends into the wider socio-political dimensions of the social world.

Now that we have some initial sense of where we are going and what we mean by humanization we shall consider in the next two chapters some of the challenges confronting integral social care and some of the most important characteristics that the integral social carer should possess.

CHAPTER FOUR

The Challenges of Integral Social Care

In this chapter I want to explore the dynamics and challenges of inter-personal integral social care in some detail. We have defined care in the previous chapters as being about the humanization of the individual through freeing them as much as is possible from personal and social oppression in order that they can exercise maximum autonomy over their own lives. The type and level of freedom each individual can enjoy depends on their particular personal and social circumstances. For example, for a person with a severe physical disability being in a position to access a shop or go to the cinema may be a huge achievement of autonomy. For an elderly person in a nursing home it may be being able to decide with other residents what type of recreational or educational services will be offered in the home. For a homeless person it may be finally gaining a flat of one's own. For some people freedom may be exercised in small steps and actions. For others it may be in bigger decisions which reshape their life.

However, for each individual, irrespective of their circumstances, the trajectory of care must be towards facilitating the person to exercise as much freedom and autonomy as possible. In this sense, to care is to bring about freedom and freedom is, in turn, not a license simply to do what one wants but the capacity and responsibility to care for oneself and others by exercising choices and making free decisions.

The question posed now is what type of characteristics and skills are required in order to equip us, the would-be carer, to be part of this process. Who is the compassionate activist? What do they look like? What do they need to know and what do they need to do?

To a large degree the answers to these questions are primarily discussed in this book in the context of the professional integral social carer. Yet I believe that the issues addressed here are of far wider implication and involve

an exploration of what it is to care more generally, how do we authentically engage in liberating relationships and even, if I may be somewhat
more presumptuous, what it is to be human. Attempting to answer these
questions amounts to a root and branch review of what we are seeking to
achieve when we practise integral care.

We have emphasized questions rather than answers. We will offer some
tentative answers but much of what is discussed here arises in the form
of key generating questions. The point is not so much to provide definitive solutions to our queries. The purpose rather is to set the direction or
orientation which may guide liberating relationships. However, by their
very nature, such relationships are open and involve the carer in engaging in a process rather than in bringing about a pre-determined outcome.
Therefore, we begin by raising some general questions to do with social
care in principle and what we mean by it before setting out some preliminary topics for consideration. Then, in the next chapter, we will suggest
seven broad areas of competence that any compassionate activist needs
to be attentive to. After all, an issue of fundamental importance is that,
before we purport to engage in intentional caring relations with another,
we need to understand who it is that we claim to be and what it is that we
think we are actually doing.

Opening questions

Therefore, before setting out to practise integral social care we can benefit from addressing a number of important preparatory questions. I have
selected six that I consider of special significance, but undoubtedly there
are others also of value that I have not addressed. There is no claim to
comprehensiveness being made here. The questions can be formulated as
follows:

1. Do we need a theory of integral social care?
2. What is the goal of integral social care?
3. What are the risks in integral social care practice?
4. What should our approach be to 'service users'?
5. How do we value what we do?
6. Who are we really in these caring relationships?

I shall take each question in turn, outlining the issue at stake and then offering a tentative initial response.

Do we need a theory of integral social care?

It is arguable that, if care is so intrinsic and fundamental to us, then social care practice should come 'naturally' to us. In this sense, we do not need to embed it in complex theories or professionalization discourses. Indeed, it could be argued that formal training and theorizing rob a certain spontaneity from the caring reflex and cause the carer to become distant from those receiving care. Through their experience of institutional education it may be that the carer becomes imbued with a new language, new concepts and new categorizations that remove him or her from the service user. These professional markers may have the effect of bestowing a new authority on the carer so that they come to consider themselves an 'expert' capable of privileged judgment over the other person. In this sense, an artificial fissure may be constructed between the category of the 'carer' and that of the 'cared-for'. I recall a manager of a major social care agency lamenting to me once that in his experience social care graduates are filled with jargon and a capacity to categorize the world, but are less capable of simply sitting down with another person and relating directly and authentically with them.

Putting this wider question in another way, we might ask whether it is necessary that a social theory should inform and shape integral social care practice. Can there be a satisfactory social care practice without a social theory? Do we need a theory to do social care work?

In a sense, of course, these questions remind us of an old and well rehearsed wider debate on the relative balance to be struck between theory and practice. The argument is that too much of one leads to too little of the other. It is clear that we cannot have practitioners whose heads are filled with theoretical understandings of social processes but who cannot simply relate personally to an oppressed human being. But neither can we have a practitioner who has little understanding of the wider social causes of poverty and exclusion. Such a practitioner would be at risk of conceptualizing care only as an interpersonal transaction orientated towards a service user with needs and deficits. They would have a naïve appreciation of contexts and settings and a limited perspective on how social problems might ultimately be addressed.

However, we must not caricature various types or styles of practice. In reality, much actual social care does occur at an interpersonal relationship level. This is perfectly understandable and appropriate. Care after all centres on authentic and liberating relationships. But, if I may offer a tentative response to the question we are here trying to address by repeating a core argument of this book, integral social care is not limited to the interpersonal domain. As we have proposed above, each individual is the product of various socio-political and cultural processes and a full understanding of the person is not achieved without an awareness of these wider factors. Thus, to truly engage in integral social care with any individual involves the carer operating at this deeper structural level also. This is the only way in which to better ensure that care is fully effective. For example, one cannot comprehensively work with a member of the Irish Travelling community without taking into account the wider social position of Travellers as an identifiable ethnic group who are subject to serious structural disadvantage. Working to care for an individual Traveller necessarily involves the compassionate activist in issues of wider socio-political concern if one wishes to genuinely provide integral care. Otherwise, the risk is that personal care takes on a benevolent, charitable hue, however unintended. The solution to private problems, whether in childcare, youth homelessness, resource allocations, and so on are often political and social rather than personal.

If integral social care is to engage with the wider social world then clearly practitioners need a thorough understanding of that world. They need to know why the social world is structured as it is, why it produces certain social problems and oppressions, and how it can be changed. They very likely need a vision of how the social world can and should be. We should not run from these challenges and hide behind an all-too-common jaded cynicism whereby we absolve ourselves of political engagement on the basis that nothing can be done.

However, integral social care should not become so orientated towards the macro perspective that it fails to see the person right before us. The person right before us takes priority. They cannot wait until we change the social world. They demand and deserve response right now. Of course, the individual also deserves that our responses are effective and that they add to our mutual humanization. Here too, we cannot avoid the responsibility of requiring a good and adequate theoretical grounding for our endeavours. In other words, we need to understand how we are to distinguish and measure humanization from dehumanization.

In short, then, the notion that there can be an effective social care practice without theoretical underpinnings is, at best, a naïve illusion and, at worst, an ideologically constructed notion designed to domesticate social care itself. Integral social care is defined by its attention both to the interpersonal dynamics of authentic and liberating relationships and to the socio-political causes of social need. Both these domains must be understood so that practice is effective. This involves combining various psychological and sociological perspectives. This book offers some suggestions in this regard and proposes one possible over-arching theoretical framework for integral social care practice. Rogers' person-centred approach will be joined with Freirean perspectives in Part Three to propose one, hopefully fruitful, theoretical combination which will centre on the notion of 'dialogic practice'. As we shall see, dialogic practice involves truly listening and responding to the person before us and acknowledging that they have the tools themselves to define and resolve the challenges confronting them.

Finally, of course both Rogers and Freire emphasize the importance of ensuring that theory is informed by practice and experience. As we have stressed above, there can be no deductive blueprint in dealing with the processes of humanization. A properly grounded theory-practice praxis should ensure that the integral social care practitioner is always reflective, critical and open to new ideas in the light of their actual experiences. A theory sealed off from experience is simply an ideology and its adherents merely closed guardians of a cult. Our rule should be – when in doubt between theory and practice, always err on the side of humanity.

What is the goal of integral social care?

This question cannot be answered unless we have some theoretical framework underpinning our social care practice. Otherwise, we are engaging in relationships with people without knowing where we want that relationship to go and why. If we do not know what we need to do in order to get to some desired destination then we have no idea in what direction we should be facing and, in the context of social care, we do not know if we are in fact causing harm rather than good.

Thus, our relationships should be purposive and orientated towards bringing about transformation. The same should be true of our socio-political concerns. They too need to be guided by a purposeful objective. The argument presented in this book is that these goals – both at an interpersonal and socio-political level – are to bring about maximum humanization, understood to mean facilitating each individual to truly become the person they want to be. A world characterized by care is one where we each support each other to be fully human.

This objective is easy to mock as idealistic and unrealizable. It may of course be extremely difficult to achieve in practice but that should not disbar us from setting it as our goal, as something we strive for and as something that provides us with the direction that allows us measure progress and civilization. If this is not our goal, then what are we prepared to say? That we wish to have a society where some can attain humanization but most cannot? That we wish for a society of winners and losers, of victors and victims? Such a society – one which we now largely have – not only is ethically abhorrent, it does not even succeed in its own terms. The Hobbesian world of each struggling for success renders everyone fearful and aggressive. It diminishes everyone.

Conceptualizing integral social care in these terms as centred on our collective humanization, where giving and receiving care are inter-changeable personal and political processes, is I think exciting and appealing. The traditional language regarding the goals of social care deployed terms such as 'normalization' and 'integration'. These terms may have implied that the individual in receipt of formal care had some form of deficit or defect which placed them outside the social norm (for which, as I've suggested before, we really mean 'average'). Therefore, the objective of care was to place them back into the 'mainstream' and, accordingly, care strategies focused on equipping them and preparing them for such integration.

Up to a point, much of this is of course well intentioned and worthy. But it carries the risk of missing certain key concerns. It assumes that the integrative difficulty lay with the individual and that the social norm itself was not in question. Yet what if the fundamental problem lay in society itself? For example, certain individuals may have a specific physical impairment but that is only a problem if society cannot accommodate such impairments. Who should change – individual or society? The disability rights movement has been able to successfully show that the disability actually rests with society not with the individual. If society is configured to accommodate all of its citizens then different physical capacities do not give rise to social exclusion. Thus, we have seen in recent years accessibility standards being adopted for all public buildings and some improvements in mobility supports in urban streets. The same issues arise for those who suffer social exclusion based on prejudice or discrimination arising from their identity, whether that be on grounds of ethnicity, race or gender.

For this reason, it is dangerous to regard the social norm as not itself potentially problematic. The social norm was once patriarchal and homophobic. Should women and gay people have been treated to 'integration' strategies so that they could adjust their expectations to the social conventions? What about slaves in nineteenth-century America? In our own time, where does the 'problem' in regards to Travellers really lie – is it with Travellers or settled society?

Thus, the discourses of normalization and integration may fail to recognize that an engagement with the excluded and oppressed should change not only them but also society itself. Dynamic mutuality requires change all around. The oppressed are not just the objects of integrative strategies, they must also be the teachers and changers of society itself. This is because, as we shall discuss below, they tell us something fundamental about the character of our society, about progress and about our common humanity.

In short, integral social care is about achieving a maximum of autonomy and freedom for each individual so that they can be, in Rogers' terms, who they really are. That is not to imply that there are no limits to freedom. Of course there are. Because we are part of a social group we must take allowance of appropriate social requirements and constraints. The issue however is where we set the standard of belonging and what type of social world we choose to construct. If we wish to include many and exclude few then that has an implication for all of us. If we wish to exclude many and include few then that creates for us a different type of society. Integral social care leads us surely to seek to include many, ideally all, in an inclusive, open community where all can find their place and all have their basic needs met. It is only in this context that many of our social problems can ultimately be resolved.

What are the risks in integral social care practice?

However, we must be cautious as we advance these claims for social transformation. As children of the twentieth century, we are wary of big ideas, particularly of big political ideas. We have seen enough of grandiose visions of political salvation, from both right and left, and seen the horrors to which they can so easily lead. Thus, we must ensure that we are considered and measured in our demands for social change and that we do not reduce our concerns to mere slogans. We use the terms considered and measured here not in the sense that we are not clear or committed but rather to avoid any suggestion that it is we alone who have all the answers to creating a humanized society. We must not elevate ourselves to be members of an enlightened elite who know exactly what we need to do. Instead we need to be open and inclusive, and mindful that integral social care practice focuses on the *process* of discovery not on assertions of pre-determined *outcomes*. This is precisely why we will emphasize the importance of engaging in a dialogic practice. Dialogue implies openness. Its opposite is monologue – where we presume to instruct others about what they ought to do.

The fact is that we do not possess any superior insight. What we do claim is that care and compassion should be at the heart of a civilized society. But, as we will outline in Chapter Eight below, the detail of such a society is open-ended, to be forged by citizens engaging together in a radically democratized process and therefore, in principle, one which is by no means predictable in advance.

As was suggested above however one of our great contemporary illusions is that we live in a society that is 'natural', that it is shaped as it is due to completely organic and inevitable causes. This is simply not true. All societies are shaped by powerful forces, such as ideas, technologies and economic and social forces. We too live under the sway of a great political idea with its attendant social and political agents moulding and forming our contemporary world. In its most recent phase we can designate it as globalization, or free-market capitalism. It is the great ideological force of our time, influencing and reaching into every aspect of our lives. It conditions our very thinking, our hopes and dreams, and determines the character of our social relations with each other. Its rules decide on the winners and losers, the included and excluded in our society. As Naomi Klein noted in her book *No Logo*,[1] this system is so all-pervasive that it has no edges; there seems to be nowhere that lies outside its embrace. For those in the Western world, this makes it strangely invisible. Because it is everywhere, like air, you no longer see it because there is no longer a place apart from it that offers sufficient contrast.

The logic of this system determines the character of our social world. The ideological principles of the system shape our values and the criteria by which we measure human success and fitness for the world. Thus we value the characteristics of competition and self-reliance and elevate for approval the actions of the self-interested rational actor. Consumerism as practice and ideal represents the epitome and marker of social success.

As we have proposed previously, the compassionate activist must of course contest this social construction on the grounds that it offers a narrow conception of the human being by diminishing the capability

[1]   N. Klein (2000), *No Logo*, London: Flamingo.

and centrality of care as a constituent and organizing principle of human sociality. But contestation should be done in a way that avoids shrillness or hectoring. Bringing care into the socio-political realm and upholding the central criterion of humanization must itself be done in a way that enhances these ends. How we act tells others about our goals and the type of world we would hope to bring about. Yes, we must be confident in our care and in our demands for social liberation but not everything is permitted to us in bringing this about. In this way we may avoid the great risk that, in our commitment to replace social indifference with social care, we too become self-appointed arbiters of what is right and wrong. Our devotion to integral social care should not lead us into a project of didactic moralization but rather inspire us to a positive project of bringing about integral humanization based on a foundation of reason, dialogue and compassion.

In similar vein, there are risks at the interpersonal level. The most obvious are that we become guilty of a form of paternalism whereby we claim that we know best. Our assertion of expertise and our very decision to engage in care, carries the risk that we position ourselves as the ones who 'know what should be done', that we are somehow qualitatively different from those receiving social care. Instead, we must remind ourselves that the single most important feature of an authentic and liberating relationship is often just to be there and to just be present with the other person. Our task then becomes not 'to know' but 'to listen' and 'to attend'. The other person is nearly always the expert in their own case. Indeed, we must remind ourselves forcibly that we will almost certainly never 'solve' anyone else's problem ourselves.

Equally we must beware of the danger of 'messianism' whereby we believe ourselves to be unique carriers of salvation. We are no such thing but the very challenges involved in integral social care, with its consequent yearnings to bring about personal and social transformation, may lead us to believe that we are the holders of a special truth not available to others. Again, as noted above, we must be modest in our caring and campaigning. We are at risk of great arrogance, and ultimately of causing disenchantment and despair to ourselves and others, if our primary motivation for integral care practice is to 'save' others and 'save' the world.

The compassionate activist must not believe that he or she is uniquely endowed with all the answers. Methodical doubt is an asset not a weakness. Human reality is more often messy and confused than not and is not readily amenable to messianic plans and commandments. We also are all too human and vulnerable to each of the vanities and weaknesses of all human beings.

Finally, there is the risk that the integral social carer uses, however unwittingly, the suffering and disadvantage of others for their own gratification, in particular to make themselves feel good or needed or important. This is a great peril and one that can easily occur. The gratitude sometimes offered by a service user, or the affirmation that is received from another, or the celebration of one's 'good works' by one's peers and friends, may become a needed motivation in maintaining one's social care practice. The danger here is that we become dependent on this affirmation so that, if we do not receive it, we become disenchanted or embittered. Worse is that receiving affirmation becomes the reason why care practice is done at all. In this case, we are *de facto* using service users for our own purposes and this is unacceptable and unethical. One of the great challenges in maintaining an authentic and liberating integral social care practice is that often there are no thanks or gratitude at all for our endeavours. This is undoubtedly a difficult aspect and one that should cause us to continually draw from our own deepest motivations and inspirations. But that is simply how it is sometimes. Service users may never acknowledge our work and our peers may well regard us as foolish or naïve and wasting our time. Whether one is praised or mocked should make little difference to the effectiveness of the work to be done. That is a tough lesson to learn but nonetheless true. We shall have more to say on this point below.

There are of course many other specific risks involved in social care. Entering into an authentic and liberating relationship is an inherently demanding task. One way to minimize or to anticipate these additional specific risks is to ensure that we are appropriately relating to all of those with whom we are in a caring relationship. This leads us to consider the next question.

What should our approach be to service users?

This question in turn brings us back to the discussion on the goals of integral social care practice. Our approach should be consistent with our goals. If we are seeking the integral liberation of the individual and are seeking to enhance their autonomy and freedom, then clearly we must work within this spirit as well. Thus there can be little place for authoritarian practice, for paternalistic superiority, for non-acceptance and judgmentalism. It is not our job at first instance to tell people what their 'problems' are or what they need to do to 'fix' them. Our job is to listen, to understand, to be present empathically and then, together, we may work jointly to achieve solutions.

For this reason, the compassionate activist should direct their work to ensuring that the *process* of the relationship is indeed authentic and liberating. The *outcome* will take care of itself and is, in any event, affected by many factors. Not least, the outcome is the responsibility in part of the service user themselves and of wider social resources and opportunities and is not the sole responsibility of the social carer. Hence, integral social carers should not judge themselves solely in accordance with measurable outcomes of 'success' or 'failure' but rather whether the relationship process they engaged in was human and respectful. That is the aspect we can take full responsibility for. But the outcome is a collective endeavour. Judging our effectiveness in terms of a pre-determined quantifiable 'target' is something that we should simply let go of. In so doing, we can relieve ourselves of much unnecessary stress. But there can be no compromise in regards to the process of the relationship.

The integral social carer therefore is a facilitator not a fixer. By non-judgmental acceptance, we can help to begin the process of liberating the person from their various personal and social oppressions. That is the most basic component of our integral care practice and something that we must take responsibility for. But, with this authentic and liberating relationship as our foundation, a variety of other social and institutional actors and resources all come into play and the effectiveness of the humanization process is the product of the interplay of all of these elements. All must be aligned for the outcome to be attained. This is why integral care refers to both the interpersonal and socio-political dimensions of the human person.

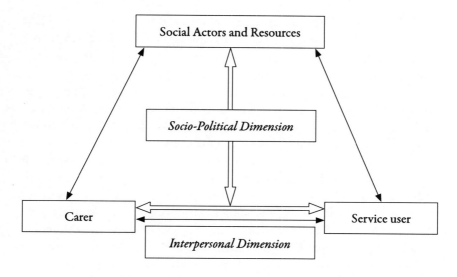

Figure One: Schema of Integral Social Care Relationship Dimensions

We need to be brutally honest about the limitations of our integral care practice in order, first, to be realistic and not naïve about what we can achieve but also, secondly, so that we do not create inflated expectations and dependency on the part of the service user. Dependency is one of the great dangers in social care work because the professional carer may appear to be the one 'who knows' and who can act purposefully compared to the receiver of care who may think of themselves as impotent and as one who 'does not know'. If this dynamic exists, it is understandable why the care receiver might hand over decision-making power to the carer. This dynamic may also be structurally reinforced by institutions of care and welfare which may explicitly conceptualize the care relationship as one between an active, knowing giver on the one hand and a passive, unknowing receiver on the other hand. Such dependency causes harm and must be carefully avoided and guarded against. It is an instrument of further oppression robbing the individual of their autonomy and agency.

That is why the *process* of care is as important as the *product*. Right from the outset of a genuine liberating relationship it must be clear that the carer is merely a facilitator – the ultimate responsibility for transformation always rests with the service user. In addition, how the person is treated – with respect, positive regard and acceptance – in itself provides a beneficial humanizing effect independently of whether the desired tangible outcome of the relationship is achieved. How people are treated has intrinsic value irrespective of the outcome of the interaction.

Of course, as noted above, this responsibility for ensuring one's own freedom is frightening and can often be resisted. This is an understandable response from people whose consciousness is oppressed by various personal and social forces. However, the integral carer must not accentuate that oppression and should instead work compassionately with the person to achieve their freedom. Many technical and therapeutic aids exist that can better help to ensure this, such as motivational interviewing, asking open questions, jointly agreeing care plans, open dialogue, anticipatory dialogue and setting in partnership achievable developmental objectives. But these are the scaffolds building the edifice. The edifice is the authentic and liberating relationship and the important point about that relationship remains that it is conducted in a dialogic process that itself must be liberating in order to attain a liberating outcome.

Finally, the process of engagement needs to be patient. Time is our great resource and indeed the only truly valuable resource there is. After all, everything else can be replaced. We must invest time in people because time is frequently required to better facilitate the humanization course. People are not machines and do not always work to timetables and short-term targets. It takes time and commitment to overcome the 'culture of silence' in which so many are sunk, a silence that prevents them expressing who they themselves are, a silence that has robbed them of their own authentic voice and view of the world. Rogers reminds us that our sense of self sometimes has to be discovered. It is not necessarily available immediately to us. It may take time, trial and error and the creativity of authentic relationships in order to excavate or uncover who we really want to be. People are rendered silent both because they have become alienated from their own true selves and also because the institutionally determined criteria of relevance and the wider ideological assumptions of our society regarding what is 'rational' and what it is to be human, can suppress their authentic voices.[2] Integral social care practice needs to be attentive to this process also and commit to a shared advocacy and authentic dialogue designed to recover the voice of those who have been made silent.

How do we value what we do?

This question naturally follows from the above. If we know what our goal is and understand the process that we must follow to achieve it, then we can appreciate what it is that we must value. We value whatever leads to humanization. The problem we have however is that this is difficult to measure in an 'objective' sense. This is in turn a problem because one of the dominant features of our contemporary society, especially within its institutional framework, is its obsession with measurement and assessment.

This obsession is the result of many factors. One is the dominance of the language and concepts of economic rationality. As was argued above, this instrumental rationality is presented as the epitome of reasonable social behaviour. Thus, actions are undertaken in the public realm if they are deemed to be efficient and to maximize measurable utility. Quantitative measurables can be modeled which allow one to demonstrate the most 'efficient' choice and that is always the one to be undertaken.

This version of instrumental rationality, initially manifested in Fordism and Taylorism, has grown in significance in the twentieth century. The American sociologist George Ritzer has coined the term 'McDonaldizaton' to describe the process in its present manifestation.[3] A McDonaldized

---

2   See in particular Foucault's *The Order of Discourse* where he outlines various 'exclusionary' devices designed to limit the production of 'rational' discourse. These include procedures of exclusion, such as prohibition, imposed standards of reason and madness and of true and false; various internal procedures; and controls over who is an acceptable speaking subject.

3   G. Ritzer (2000), *The McDonaldization of Society*, Thousand Oaks, CA: Pine Forge Press.

system is one which is guided by the imperatives of efficiency (understood in instrumental-rational terms), predictability, calculability and control (especially of variable elements such as people). Further impetus for this mindset occurred in the 1980s following the elections of Margaret Thatcher and Ronald Reagan. The decision to reform social welfare systems and to demonstrate public service 'performance' according to newly constructed criteria, gave rise to the creation of a whole series of 'objective' measurables designed to demonstrate efficiency in these hitherto non-marketized domains. This in turn gave rise to a new 'managerialism', based on notions of ensuring the application of free market rationality into public service provision. Wide powers were granted from the 1980s onwards to a new cadre of managers which had the result of limiting the power and autonomy of other professionals and subjecting them to new performance management systems. Thus, there emerged increased centralized regulation of work processes, output-based targets and financing and a gradual but inexorable replacement of the ethos of personal service work by mechanical and systematic practices.

Under this system the manager decides and the employee obeys. A culture of mistrust is created whereby any autonomy exercised by the individual worker is suspect and therefore subjected to new forms of monitoring and regularization.

This regime has had a catastrophic impact on contemporary social care practice as well as on many other fields. It takes little account of the time–rich context within which liberating relationships must occur. Indeed, it seeks specifically to re-orient social care towards performance indicators which often have little real connection to the human needs of service users.

This is precisely why we need absolute clarity regarding what is of real value in integral social care. Many of the indicators developed as part of the performance management ideology need to be contested and abandoned. They have no place in integral social care and serve now only to justify the role of a management cadre that often adds little real value to the work to be done.

The danger is that these measurables orient practice away from what is important and onto what is far less valuable but more easily demonstrable.

All too often I have heard experienced practitioners lament their attention being diverted onto trivial (but measurable) matters at the expense of work that was of far greater genuine value.[4] Far more importantly, the service users themselves know what counts and what does not. It is they who are the only true determiners of the effectiveness of integral care practice. Yet often their wishes too are made subservient to the prescribed tasks or plans set out for them.

In this sense, the notion of 'person-centred' care has become largely a pious aspiration, existing only as a virtuous declaration of value contained in a wide range of official statements of intention and policies. Every organization is 'person-centred' in aspiration but, in reality, person-centred practice does not lend itself to performance measurement. Instead, fixed menus of service provision, efficient 'streamlining' of services and deductive plans based on available resources have all served to contract actual delivery to a predetermined, McDonaldized version of provision. Time – that most important of all resources – has become measured, rationed and controlled. The setting for authentic relationship-building has been contracted.

We need to recover a shared vision of what is valuable in integral social care. As professionals, integral social care workers need to assert where the true value of social care lies. We need to affirm what is genuinely important in our work. Every plan and every system should be subject to the core value of whether it enhances or diminishes the humanization of each particular person that is being engaged with. That is the only true value. The arbiter of that humanization is the individual person themselves. If this is

---

4   Examples of this include the care worker who is too busy with prescribed, allocated tasks to have a conversation with a service user. The worker is obliged to follow not their own judgement but the prescribed schedule of tasks which will later be checked and recorded. Consider also the notorious example of the *de facto* forced feeding of an elderly person in their home by a home care worker because this is a prescribed task which must be performed even if the elderly person indicates that they do not wish to eat at that time. The worker feels obliged to ensure that the feeding has occurred in order to comply with the pre-determined care regime which must be accomplished, most likely within the limited timeframe of the home visit itself. The worker avoids exercising a professional judgement in favour of adherence to the plan even if this results in a dehumanizing interaction with the elderly person.

not central to our practice then we may well be busy and 'efficient' but we are not necessarily effective. Effectiveness and efficiency are not the same thing. As Ritzer argues compellingly, too much efficiency, predictability, calculability and control ultimately defeats its own purpose and gives rise to dehumanization.[5]

In integral social care there is no neutrality. Either we are for humanity or against it. Blind obedience to a system is not in itself a virtue. As we have already suggested, if in doubt we must always err on the side of humanity.

Who are we in these relationships?

In our social care relationships, then, what stance do we take? Do we reproduce oppression, even if unwittingly, or challenge it and facilitate liberation? Is the contemporary social carer to assume the role of a detached professional and be the dispenser of solutions based on claims to expertise? In what precise role do we present ourselves before the people we wish to work with?

All that has been argued thus far in this book suggests that above all we must think of ourselves primarily as human beings involved in an authentic liberating relationship. *We meet our service users on the plain of our common humanity.* There is no qualitative or ontological difference between us. We are all interchangeably givers and receivers of care. This implies that our overwhelming tendency to judge and categorize – both ourselves and others – must, at first instance, be set aside. Conceptualizing our work through categories and labels, whether that be of professional / expert on the one side or that of customer / client on the other, only get in the way. They interpose between a subject-to-subject authentic relationship by implicitly introducing hierarchies of power and privileged knowledge.

---

5   For example, it may be efficient to drive a car from A to B because this is the quick-
est and easiest way to make the journey. But if everyone drives then the road will be
clogged and no-one will make the journey quickly. Equally, it may be efficient to
eat at a fast-food restaurant rather than cook at home but if that is all you do then
your health will ultimately be compromised.

These do not help initially. They accentuate the marginalization of the service user and may add, however unintended it might be, to their experience of oppression.

True non-judgmental acceptance occurs when we permit ourselves to be a person and see the other as a person also. It is the recognition of our common humanity that permits us to have an empathic response to the experience of the other. In empathy, our human experience (limited as it may well be) reaches out to the other's human experience (extreme as it may be). Our experiences of anger, of hurt, of exclusion, of oppression and of dependence can lead us to a better understanding of their experiences of these things. If we are not open to this mutuality – this shared interchange of experience and feelings – then we are opting for a subject-object relationship. In that case we are hiding ourselves behind our own professional mask and can only appear to the other person as someone detached and only half present.

The compassionate activist should not fear, or flee from, their own feelings. It is these feelings that maintain our humanity and better help us to avoid coldness or burn-out. In most social care relationships, two important 'transactions' are going on. First, there is the actual service or resource that the service user is seeking. This could be a physical support, a benefit or allowance of some kind or a service of some sort. These can be achieved or not and can be achieved slowly or not.[6] All integral social care strives for effectiveness at this level. But, second, there is also the interpersonal exchange. This is the exchange of mutuality, of respect and of acceptance. Was the person enhanced in their humanity or, through their interaction with the social carer, in any way diminished? Often, the physical resources sought cannot be achieved. This is a failure but one that almost always is outside the power of the carer to secure. But the carer is responsible for the manner of their relationship with the service user. Here, there should be no failure. No service user should ever leave with their humanity diminished. The compassionate activist never compromises on this crucial aspect. We

6   This is the level largely determined by political choices regarding resource allocations and service prioritizations.

may be ineffective in regards to the tangible service resource but must never be in regards to our relationships. If integral social care is focused on enhancing humanization, then that begins immediately in our mutual encounter with the other person.

However, there are crucial limits to what can be done. Knowing what these limits are is important in order to preserve the effectiveness of the relationship exchange. The social carer must also preserve their humanity and their capacity to persevere and be effective. This necessarily involves a recognition that there must be boundaries to any relationship. This recognition of course is not just a feature of social care relationships. These should not be pathologized as though they were some kind of unique sub-set of 'normal' relationships. *All* our relationships have certain boundaries. Knowing what is appropriate to say and not to say, understanding rules of etiquette and courtesy, preserving conventions regarding touch, sexuality, aggression and so on are boundaries built in to every relationship. Every human relationship operates within a structured framework of what is reasonable and appropriate to do or say. It is often breaches of this implied framework that leads to relationships breaking down.

It is precisely to avoid this that we need to be mindful of the specific boundaries required in integral social care. Boundaries serve to protect the relationship. There must be limits in any relationship and social care relationships are no different. The specific boundaries that are required are determined by the specificities of each relationship and cannot be simply pre-determined. This issue will be treated in somewhat more detail in the following chapter.

Finally, being involved in a real and authentic relationship means that we may on occasion challenge or confront the other. But this too should not be regarded as unique to social care. In all our relationships – if they are real and secure – we should be able to confront. Any relationship that only permits agreement and acquiescence is one that is in reality fragile. Challenging occurs once we have a secure relationship based on mutual trust and non-judgemental acceptance. Then, a challenge or confrontation is the act of someone who cares, who wishes the other well. It is not the act of one who judges. This is a complex and subtle dynamic requiring great discernment and wisdom. The moment in a social care relationship where the carer says 'no' to the service user, or says to him/her 'you should not do this' is a defining moment when, if the foundation is strong, leads the relationship to new depth. But this word of challenge can only be sounded in a setting of respect and acceptance. Only in this setting can the word of challenge be humanizing rather than oppressive.

In short, the integral social carer should be themselves in their social care relationships. Who else could they be? Why be someone else? If they strive to act a role as 'carer', or 'professional', then they will undermine the human mutuality of the relationship. However, ensuring that they present and behave appropriately in the social care relationship is no different in principle to how they must act in every relationship they have. Tempering one's reactions, refraining from critical responses and remaining calm and tolerant are all aspects which feature in any meaningful relationship that one has. Maintaining these conventions does not make one inauthentic. They are merely the requirements of any respectful human interaction. Authenticity is determined in you being yourself, not acting out a role, and truly engaging with the other's frame of reference while being fully aware of your own experiences and feelings in the relationship. As is appropriate in any unfolding relationship, your feelings will inevitably be expressed or manifested in due course. But first, the authentic integral carer chooses to really listen and pay attention to the other person and opens themselves to the possibility that they will be moved by the other and perhaps even changed. If we are hiding behind a mask or a self-constructed role then this is unlikely to happen. Indeed the mask is designed to ensure that it will not happen.

Tentative propositions or provocations

The preliminary opening questions outlined above introduce us to some of the big concerns in contemporary professional practice. However, as I have proposed throughout this text, the issues raised here are not just pertinent to professional practitioners. All citizens may be engaged in integral social care at one level or another. In order therefore to expand our reflection on integral care, I propose now to set out a series of propositions regarding care that I consider to have application in many settings, whether professional or not. Despite the declarative character of these propositions, I mean them to be quite tentative statements that might serve to guide effective practice. Many of them have the ring of exhortations but, despite the risk of sanctimoniousness, all of them are designed to provoke a response and stimulate debate and discussion. I make no claim to originality here. Most of these ideas are well understood in the social care literature. Nor do I make a claim to comprehensiveness. Many additional issues of importance are undoubtedly not addressed here. Therefore, this is merely *one* possible set of propositions out of many possible sets. These propositions are presented from the perspective of the social carer because, after all, reflection on their specific role is the purpose of this book. Hence, the somewhat exclusive terminology used is frequently that of 'we' and 'the other person'.

Integral social care occurs in an authentic and liberating relationship

Enough has been said about this proposition in this book without need for further repetition. Suffice it to say that integral care must begin within mutual relationships characterized by authenticity and orientated towards the humanization of each party through a process of mutual liberation. This liberation is both personal and social. Its precise character and the precise form humanization takes, depends on the specific oppression that the individual suffers from. A physical disability, a psychological difficulty or a social prejudice, confer different oppressions and require different responses. Nonetheless, in virtually all cases, humanization and hence compassionate activism requires both interpersonal and socio-political responses. All problems are likely to be both personal and social. Their specific configuration will determine the particular caring response. However, while integral care looks to all dimensions of the human person it must be grounded in the individual human person who stands before us and in a relationship to that unique and valuable person.

Integral social care begins with me

The authentic interpersonal relationship begins with me because I am responsible for my own authenticity. I cannot determine the authenticity of the other person but I can ensure that, in the relationship, I am who I am and by virtue of that acceptance of myself encourage the other to be themselves also. Me being me allows you to be you. To put this in the Rogerian terms discussed in Chapter Two, I must ensure that I am open to experience, that I trust in my own feelings and ideas, that I cultivate an internal locus of evaluation and that I am open to change. Thus, I enter a social care relationship open to the possibility (the inevitability?) that I will change as a result of these interactions.

In addition, I must ensure that I have the right disposition for integral care, particularly an orientation towards non-judgmental acceptance and humanization. The point here is that we should not begin from a focus on fixing the other person. We begin with ourselves and ensure that we are correctly and effectively orientated and disposed towards the other. We begin with ourselves not for our sake but for the sake of the other person. In part also, a positive orientation towards the other also means allowing ourselves to be compassionate and freeing ourselves from the false notion that we should only look after our own interests.

Authentic integral social care begins now

Commitment to integral care and compassionate activism begins now in our immediate circumstances. It is a contradiction in terms to claim to care about various categories of oppressed people and various causes if one exercises limited care within one's existing social networks, particularly those of one's immediate family. The test as to whether you are really committed to a practice of care is your own family and your own immediate circle of work mates, companions and community. Bring care home! Make it real today right where you are. Care should not be conceptualized in abstracted terms as pertaining only to one's relationship to specific people in specific circumstances. We have had enough of ideologues and false saints whose outward image is one of caring but who are neglectful and indifferent within their own domestic worlds. The best preparation for professional care practice or for a more general commitment to compassionate activism is at home. The best measure of one's authenticity to this commitment is how one treats those in one's own home. The best way to create a civilization of care is to begin here and now with those whom we daily encounter.

You are you and they are they

Despite our convictions and compassion we must not forget that we are not the other person. Our compassion for another person must not be such as to cause us to lose our own personal identity. While empathy can take us close to the feelings of the other, and acceptance bring us close to their perspective, we can never become the other person. We can never fully enter their experiences. It is naïve and potentially dangerous to believe that we can. We cannot become them and we cannot live their lives. Authentic relationships grounded on acceptance and mutuality only works on the basis that we recognize the intrinsic value and identity of *each* subject in the relationship and that includes us. Thinking that we can merge both subjects into one is a gross error and gives rise to fundamental dysfunctions such as dependency whereby the other person becomes an adjunct of the carer or the carer becomes utterly reliant on the needs or affirmation of the other. In short, identities must always be preserved.

The other person is not there to meet your needs

It is a cardinal ethical principle that the other person is not there to serve us. They are not objects whose value lies in their benefit to us. They cannot be used for our personal purposes. This principle, while clear in theory, can in fact be breached in complex and subtle ways. For example, it is possible that people drawn into social care work may, in order to feel of value, need to be needed or need to be liked and praised by others. Entering into relationships with vulnerable people may become a cheap and easy way for us to be liked and needed as persons.

The integral social carer must be very careful here. The sufferings of others should not be the ground of our happiness. Otherwise, we can develop an improper, although often unrecognized, vested interest in the continuation of their suffering rather than in their liberation. Neither should we seek advantage from the sufferings of another by seeking to derive some public value or approval from our work with the oppressed and marginalized. As we have noted above, the danger here is that the carer may come to need and become dependent on the social affirmation that arises. The risk is that without this approval we may become de-motivated. Compassionate activism should never be undertaken for applause. In short, apart from the obvious wrong in overtly using another person for our own ends in any way whatsoever, we should not use our engagement with the oppressed in order to secure subtle benefits for ourselves, whether they be personal, social or religious.

Only the other person can live their own life and be the author of their own solutions

Recognizing the integrity and intrinsic value of the other person should place a natural limit on the practice and actions of the integral social carer. The other person's life is their life. They must live it as they choose. The carer must let go of their natural tendency to evaluate and propose solutions. The carer must not become an intrusive, judgmental and interventionist force. A person-centred approach dictates that the other person is always the author of their own life and choices. The social carer is a facilitator, a supporter, an advocate, a dialogue partner and should not imagine themselves to be in the role of a parent to a child or to be an enlightened 'fixer' of the other person's problems. Their suggestions and ideas should be offered, when invited, in a spirit of dialogue. The other person should always be regarded as the expert on their own situation and on the 'solutions' that are appropriate to them. This is because the other person is nearly always the best judge of their own needs. The integral social carer should beware the temptation towards exercising expertise and *de facto* power over the other. Better to listen, to learn and to support rather than to instruct, to dictate and to decide.

In truth, liberating relationships involve a reciprocal exchange within which the *bona fide* knowledge of the carer may well be of value and assistance. But this should be offered in a spirit of suggestion and facilitation. After all, only the other person knows the full facts and circumstances of their own lives. The carer intervenes and meddles in that complexity only with great caution and respect.

In integral social care, time and presence are the most important resources of all

The greatest offering that the social carer makes is that of their own time. Time is the soil from which relationships grow. The giving of time is a tangible sign of commitment and acceptance. Identifying time as the most important resource places the emphasis on presence, on 'being there', and points to the non-dramatic, mundane character of authentic social care relationships. There should be no drama in our relationships. Rather they should be stable and secure and measured in their effectiveness by the extent to which we can abide calmly and tolerantly with each other. Other 'therapeutic' skills often associated with social care may have a superficial allure about them but 'being present' is the most significant of all. This is the commitment to be beside another person, to accompany them and to listen to them. The concern in this emphasis is not so much on performing certain pre-set objectives, important as they may be. It is rather on ensuring a relationship based on acceptance and oriented towards personal and social liberation. By not giving the necessary time to this, the social carer is implicitly not valuing the being and rhythms of another person and this merely adds to the sum of oppression. The resilience and commitment of the integral carer is truly tested and revealed when despite being rejected, or shouted at, or ignored they remain present and open to the other person's experiences and communication. In contemporary professional social care practice the combination of a lack of resources and a flawed emphasis on certain performance indicators has eroded the valuing and availability of time to the point where much social care is now a rush of activity resulting only in stress and dehumanization for both carer and service user alike.

The focus should be on process not product

As has been emphasized above, integral social care focuses on the process of humanization within an authentic and liberating relationship. The carer can take responsibility for that process by ensuring that it is grounded in non-judgmental acceptance. But humanization is open-ended. It cannot in principle be defined or measured in advance. We cannot know deductively how we become ourselves. It is uncovered and discovered in the dynamics of our relationships and in the exercise of our free choices. Thus, the 'product' of our relationships must take care of itself. Equally, this 'product' is the responsibility of the other person. The carer can only engage authentically in the process of relationship but they cannot determine its result and should therefore not look to 'end products' to measure their 'success'. Too many variables and too many decisions by others determine that final destination. The carer can only attend to the process unfolding in the present moment.

Relationships are a moral enterprise

All relationships with human beings are moral enterprises. As argued above, we must not turn people into objects either in our treatment of them or in our use of them. Our attitude and disposition towards the other person must be governed by the principle of intrinsic value. The other person is valuable now, exactly as they are and not just as they might become in the future. Their value does not lie in their personal usefulness or in their wider social utility. A person who becomes a paraplegic or otherwise disabled or marginalized remains a person with intrinsic value. Genuine relationships are those of a subject to subject, characterized by mutuality and acceptance.

In a Western society so centred on commodification[7] such as ours we can easily come to regard human beings themselves as commodities and of value only insofar as they possess economic utility.

In many Western societies, Ireland prominent among them, we have witnessed in recent years a disturbing ethical collapse within the institutions of public governance and service. Many public bodies and individuals in positions of responsibility have been shown to have treated people as objects to be lied to, to be cheated and to be abused in a variety of ways. The *Ryan Report* into institutional sexual abuse, the *Honohan Report* into the banks and the prison visiting committee reports into Mountjoy Prison all reveal fundamental moral failure as well as other procedural failures. Even (maybe especially) when working within institutional settings, the compassionate activist must never lose their personal moral autonomy. We are always moral agents who should act accordingly. Following orders, or hiding behind the corporate 'culture', are no justifications for treating people as though they were objects. We shall discuss in the next chapter the fundamental ethical principle of doing no harm to another person.

Avoid creating dependency

This is a proposition of great importance and has been briefly discussed already. It is one of the more obvious and known risks in social care that the other person may become dependent on the carer. The carer is in a positive and affirming relationship with them, has accepted them and seems to have knowledge and competence. For many people who are at points of great vulnerability this may be an overwhelming experience. As a result, they may feel themselves to be in the process of becoming a person perhaps for the first time. In this circumstance, it is understand-

---

7   By commodification is meant the phenomenon by which items are valued according to their monetary sale value.

able that a close bond may be forged. The great danger in this dynamic, of course, is if they make the carer the source and conduit of their own well-being and of their own happiness. They may come to feel that their happiness rests on the carer.

These feelings of positive reliance and regard may prove very powerful for the carer also and may lock the carer into a different type of dependency, as discussed above, whereby their sense of worth is tied into the affirmation received. Great attention is needed at this point. It is so important that the integral carer is focused on the purpose and meaning of the relationship as one centred on the liberation and humanization of the other person. This may mean letting go, learning to say no and learning to step back from the other person. The great challenge and difficulty in integral social care is finding on each occasion the balance between acceptance and mutuality on the one hand and facilitation and liberation on the other. There is no manual for this as each human being and each situation is unique. What is required is sound judgment, good support and wisdom. In this sense, the integral carer must learn when and how to let go the bonds of dependency between him/her and the service user. The carer must recognize that they cannot and should not control everything. On the contrary, power must be held by the other person to the maximum extent possible in the circumstances. The integral carer must be clear from the outset that the other person is the author of their own life. They must be open about their own limits and weaknesses and the limits of the relationship. An old maxim is never to promise what you cannot deliver.

The hard reality and peculiar paradox of social care relationships is that they may end precisely at the point where the other person has begun the process of liberation. While they are oppressed and requiring support the relationship proceeds but when the other reaches a point of autonomy the relationship may need to be let go (or at least radically reframed). The danger is that both parties fear taking this step each for their own reasons. But it must be taken in a spirit of genuine compassion and commitment to the humanization of each.

Maintain a joyful mind

To be blunt, much nonsense is written about the power of positive think-ing. It is as if the horrors and trials of the world can be made invisible if we only think positive thoughts. However, if we can leave aside this sim-plistic presentation of the issue, there is nonetheless little doubt that those with a joyful and peaceful mind tend to experience life joyfully, even in the midst of pain. The philosopher Wittgenstein famously noted that the happy person lives in a happy world and, adapting this insight somewhat, the novelist Iris Murdoch argued that the good person literally lives in a different world to that of the bad person. Long before either of them, the great English poet John Milton wrote in *Paradise Lost*, Book I, 'The mind is its own place and of itself can make a heaven of hell, a hell of heaven'. Prior to Milton, the Buddhist tradition developed ideas and techniques of great depth and insight into how and why one might maintain a peaceful, calm and happy mind. For Buddhism, our happiness cannot rest on outer conditions because these continually change and are not under our control. Therefore, happiness must be the product of inner conditions, specifically how our mind reacts to the vagaries and circumstances of life. For this reason, the various Buddhist schools have formulated diverse methods for training the mind to be calm and peaceful.

These ideas will be further explored below but for now it can also be noted that, for complex psychological reasons, the happiness and peaceful-ness we exhibit can be transmitted to another. Thus, maintaining a joyful mind is not just an issue for us personally, in terms of our own health and well-being. In fact there is little doubt that we are affected by, and in turn effect, the disposition and emotions of another. Emotions and feelings are transferred between us through the varied and highly sophisticated reper-toire of human interpersonal communication. Thus, those with a happy mind do indeed tend to create or encourage happiness about them. They draw out the happiness in the other. Those with stress and anger tend to inspire similar feelings in others. That we are profoundly affected by the feelings of others is a basic social-psychological assumption. There is a fundamental reciprocity in human interactions. If I treat someone well the chances are that they will respond in kind. If I treat them badly then I should expect the same in return.

For these reasons, cultivating a happy mind, and giving ourselves permission to maintain a happy mind, is a critical advantage in entering into authentic and liberating relationships. Positive inner dispositions are likely to create positive outer reactions. As we shall see below, one of the key characteristics of the compassionate activist is that he or she acts with a mind of love and care and not from one of hatred and anger. After all, as we intuitively know, love attracts and hate repels. Without love there can be no humanization.

Conflict is a feature of all social groups: accept it and do not run from it

To balance however what has just been stated, we need also to recognize that all social groups are characterized by conflict. At the very least there is invariably conflict over scarce resources, whether these are material or symbolic. In any group, large or small, there tends also to be inevitable conflict over status. Conflict is simply another inherent aspect of our sociality. This is important to recognize because it means that we can never attain a condition where *all* conflict is eliminated. That is not possible. Our very sociality commits us to mutual dependency and reliance on others and therefore, in situations where our needs are not fulfilled, conflict is an inevitable consequence. Human beings themselves are often needy and demanding. Most of our relationships have some element of ambiguity built into them. There are almost always aspects of other people – even those we love – that we struggle to accept or find difficult to like. In addition, the order of human relations and hierarchies are always contestable.

Thus, conflict is 'normal'. No amount of positive thinking will get rid of it but having peaceful minds will better permit us to manage it and de-escalate it rather than accentuate it. The point here is that the integral social carer must be prepared and able for conflict. It must not frighten or disable them so that they cannot deal with it. They must have a realistic understanding of the social world and of the people in it. The issue then is not whether they can eliminate it but whether by their actions and words the integral social carer adds to the sum of conflict or reduces it.

The service users that they will most likely encounter are often themselves the victims and losers of interpersonal and social conflict and this can add to their vulnerability and defensiveness with others. Displays of aggression and anger can often mask weakness and fear. Violence is conflict brought to an extreme. In instances where the integral carer experiences violence their task is to always attempt to de-escalate it and to never add to violence or anger. There are many well-tried techniques that can be learned to do this which can be gleaned from other books and manuals. Describing these however is beyond the scope of this book.

In short, conflict should not be regarded necessarily as an aberration or a dysfunction.[8] It is an intrinsic part of the human reality and, if manifested in violence, should be paid attention to on the grounds that it is telling us something about the person involved and their social circumstances. Violence, however horrific and upsetting, is a form of communication. This is by no means to excuse violence. On the contrary, violence is the ultimate manifestation of oppression and it should be understood in that context. However, the compassionate activist should not have an innocent or naïve conception of the social world as one where reason and good arguments always succeed. Any intervention in that world designed to bring about transformation almost inevitably leads to conflict at some level. The compassionate activist needs therefore to be aware and prepared for this and not daunted in their endeavours. We must be assertive and committed to our own beliefs and values and be prepared to defend and manifest them in our integral care practice.

8   For an interesting study of this point see Felix O'Murchadha (ed.) (2006), *Violence, Victims, Justifications: Philosophical Approaches*, Bern: Peter Lang AG.

Campaigning is part of caring

Finally, leading on from these observations, it can be seen how integral social care must not avoid the burdens and challenges of campaigning, of advocacy and of politics. This is because, as noted in the Introduction above and elsewhere in this book, marginalization and oppression, while made visible at a personal level, more than often have their causes in the social and political dimensions. At the most basic level, campaigning is frequently required in order to secure appropriate resource allocations and priority. Getting these to those who truly need them often demands overt political activism. However, at a more fundamental and complex level, it is primarily the structures of society that produce poverty and exclusion in the first place. These problems, whether they be for example unemployment, homelessness or anti-social behaviour, which manifest themselves at a personal level, cannot be solved unless we attend to their political causes. The integral social carer is identified by his or her commitment to these socio-political dimensions as well as to the interpersonal dimensions of care. Thus, I think it entirely appropriate that the integral carer is inspired by a vision of a just and equal society and world in which care for all can better be structurally realized and in which, at the very least, the basic needs of all to food, shelter and education can be met. In this sense, compassionate activism is concerned with social justice and equality and chooses to consciously act within the political domain. In our world today, for care to be effective it must be political.

The challenges and propositions outlined in this chapter are certainly formidable. However, by identifying and recognizing them, we gain I believe an insight into the personal and professional characteristics required from the integral social carer. The next chapter proceeds to examine these in more detail.

CHAPTER FIVE

The Characteristics of the Integral Social Carer

Having addressed a number of general opening questions and a series of propositions designed to stimulate debate, I want now to progress our reflections by briefly outlining seven core competencies or characteristics to which the integral social carer requires to be attentive. Once again, I make no claim to either originality or comprehensiveness. There may be other competencies that I have neglected here which perhaps might be equally highlighted. Certainly, there are crucial issues pertaining to contemporary social care which I have not addressed such as questions of resource deficits and their impact on care provision, pay and conditions, the adequacy of training and education, the quality of social care management, poor institutional support and the complex regulatory and legal framework surrounding social care provision. However, these are issues that have been well addressed in other publications. In this book, the competencies to be explored are better considered to be general domains and thematic concerns that need to be considered as part of any theory or conception of integral social care. To some extent they repeat and build on the various initial observations made in the previous chapter. In summary, they are:

- The Self
- Compassion
- Boundaries
- Communication
- Ethics
- Knowledge
- Technical Skills

I shall address some of these areas in greater detail than others, as explained below.

The self

Integral social care begins with the self. This proposition has been discussed above. However, this essential idea bears repetition. It does so because, if integral social care is conceptualized at first instance as an authentic and liberating relationship with another, then we need to know exactly who we are in that relationship. We need to know this because the instrument we are deploying into that care dynamic is not a set of tools or even techniques. It is primarily our very selves as persons. Therefore, it is critical that our selves are properly grounded and secure, are orientated correctly in terms of values and understandings, and are prepared sufficiently so that we are effective in our care. A key assumption being made here is that the self is not fixed and determined but fluid and open to change.

There are two aspects to this readying of self. First, there must be self-knowledge whereby I know who I am as a person who is in a continual process of becoming, know my strengths and weaknesses, know my limits, and know my motivations for engaging in social care relationships. Second, there must be self-care whereby I ensure that I have compassion for myself, that I care for myself and that I am enhancing my own humanization. In summary, we must start with the self in order to better ensure that I am not an agent of dehumanization either for the other person or for myself. Let us take each dimension in turn.

Self-knowledge

In authentic social care relationships (probably indeed in all authentic relationships) the person we most encounter is ourselves. If we are genuinely open to our experiences then it is we who are revealed to ourselves. Our strengths, our capacities, our weaknesses and our vulnerabilities are laid bare in the dynamic of a genuine relationship. We can of course choose to ignore these revelations and hide behind our masks or we can choose to face them and attend to them in an ongoing process of discovery.

The more we know of ourselves the better prepared we are for the encounter with the other person. In our mutual exchange with the other, especially if it is characterized by honesty and compassion, our common humanity is revealed. The more we know of ourselves, the more we can know the other. Indeed, I must know myself in order to know another. If I am blind in regards to myself, the chances are that I will be blind in regards to the other also. I must accept myself as I really am in order to accept the other as he or she really is.

I must find in myself what I see in the other. The oppression in him/her is in me too. The suffering in him/her is in me too. The longing for liberation and humanization in him/her is in me too. The extent and depth of these may well be of completely different orders of course but I must not pretend that I too do not have all the human range of feelings and hurts and desires that he/she has. Recognizing that in me too can be found this shared repository of human experiences is crucial in order that there can be empathy and understanding. It is the acknowledgment of this commonality that permits acceptance and builds genuine compassion.

Developing self-knowledge is about being fully open to our experiences. We should not filter them or judge them as unacceptable. Rather we should set aside the idealized versions of ourselves and experience each moment to the fullest. We need to become alert to what is happening about us and engage in a form of deep seeing. We need to pay attention and to wake up to the immediate. Our best learning is found in responding to whatever is happening to us at this very instant.[1]

This is not about self-absorption. It is only by accepting ourselves that we can accept others. Otherwise, it is often the case that what we hate and reject in others are actually aspects of ourselves. We project blame and rejection outward in order to get it away from ourselves. Problems are then someone else's fault. This tendency to shift blame and condemnation onto others rather than ourselves can also occur at the wider, social level. Thus it is easier, in order to maintain our comfortable lifestyle, to blame

---

[1] For some very interesting reflections on this subject see Pema Chödrön (2001), *When Things Fall Apart: Heart Advice for Difficult Times*, Boston: Shambhala.

the poor for their poverty and to ascribe their deprivation to laziness or some other moral defect on their part. Therefore, if we want to awaken compassion we can do this by awakening compassion for ourselves first. Knowing my own failures and needs and humanity does not lead me into self-centredness in a narrow sense. Instead, if it is genuine, it leads me into recognizing the same failures, needs and humanity in the other. His fears are my fears, her tears are my tears.

Finally, the compassionate activist strives not only for personal congruence, to use Rogers' term once more, but also seeks to ensure that all of his or her actions are done with one intention – to manifest care in order to liberate the other. In a general, intuitive manner, we know that more often than not if we act negatively it leads to negativity but if we act positively it leads to the positive. This is the route not just to our own humanization but also to the humanization of the other person. If this is so, then we have almost stumbled upon an (admittedly unprovable!) claim of what is the good, fulfilled and meaningful life – *to be fully aware of the present moment and to fill that moment with maximum compassion*. This may amount to a statement of the meaning and purpose of life, unverifiable of course in its saying but compelling in its living.

Self-care

Yet this self is fragile and vulnerable. The encounter with human suffering and oppression imposes huge physical and psychological demands. The self must be protected and nurtured and not thrown lightly into integral care practice. If our self is damaged in this practice then this is of little benefit to us and little benefit to the other person.

How then is the self to be protected and nurtured? Part of this is achieved when we have a good understanding of the self. This involves being aware of what we are experiencing and being able to articulate that awareness to ourselves and others. It involves awareness of one's weaknesses and vulnerabilities so that one knows when to pause, to take stock, to rest and to withdraw. It involves developing an internal locus of evaluation so that one is not buffeted by the judgments of others. It involves recognizing the limits of one's role and that one is not responsible alone for the outcome of relationships. Recognition of the limits of one's role also allows us recognize the boundaries and institutional frameworks within which professional practice must operate.

For the professional social care worker, it is crucial that they acknowledge that they are not their work. Their self is not limited to, or defined by, their work. This must be the case with all of us in all of our varied circumstances – *we are not our work*. If work is allowed to define us then our well-being and happiness are determined by forces outside our control and this is oppressive. Self-care then must centre on ensuring our personal liberation from various oppressions.

Key to this is maintaining a wide range of relationships which we cultivate continually. The compassionate activist too needs care and needs to ensure that their own networks of support and encouragement are maintained. Time-out, relaxation, physical exercise and a certain detachment from outcomes (not from process) all form components of self-care. We should never become dependent on an outcome that we cannot control. For this reason we must enter into our social care relationships somewhat disarmed – disarmed of our superiority and of our power to determine results as we want them to be.

Finally, I think we can care for ourselves by enhancing our own humanization through cultivating compassionate change in ourselves. This process of transformation of the self should be a key project of the compassionate activist. That the self is open to continual change and that we can engage in a process of self-transformation through the choices we make is a profound idea which is central to much contemporary psychology and modern existentialist philosophy. But this is not a new idea. As has been shown above, most cultures have constructed idealized versions of the human being which is offered as a model for meaningful living. Virtually all of the great religions in a variety of cultures have proposed normative models for human life. Of particular interest in this regard has been the Western world's recent engagement with Buddhism. As has been acknowledged above, Buddhism's two-and-a-half thousand years of reflection on this very process of personal transformation offers us empirically verifiable and viable ways to accomplish such a compassionate change in oneself.

Irrespective of its wider metaphysical or religious claims (which for our purposes can be set to one side) Buddhism provides us with one possible set of methodologies for such transformations.

In engaging with this method or process we can begin by acknowledging that each of us are full of positive and negative emotions and feelings which manifest themselves in positive and negative actions. The positive emotions include compassion, patience and a desire to do no harm to another. The negative include anger, hatred and rejection. We might also acknowledge, as has been argued above, that positive emotions and actions are more likely to lead to personal happiness. This is surely self-evident. We all feel happier being surrounded by, and experiencing, love rather than hatred.

We need therefore to become mindful of our emotions and actions. We need to pay close attention to whether we generally act positively or negatively. In particular, we should become mindful of our habitual responses. What do we automatically do when angry, when hurt, when frightened? When do we have these emotions and why? With this mindfulness, we can then consciously cultivate positive emotions and actions. We can challenge our habitual responses and seek, in Mattieu Ricard's rich phrase, through a 'dialogue with the emotions', to let go the negative emotions and replace them with the positive.[2] If we advance in this practice we can gain sufficient insight and control to observe our own emerging emotions and say to ourselves 'this is me becoming angry!' and choose to let it go. Of course, this degree of self-awareness and control is extremely difficult to achieve but it surely forms the defining trajectory of the process of humanization. If we want others to be positive and happy then why not ensure it for ourselves first?

Cultivating and developing this level of mindfulness is undoubtedly a lifetime project. Mindfulness can be enhanced by our willingness to dwell in the present moment, to pay attention to what is happening about us and in us, and through speaking and listening with compassion.

2   For further reference see Mattieu Ricard (2006), *Happiness: A Guide to Developing Life's Most Important Skill*, New York: Little, Brown and Company.

Calm and deep breathing, slow purposeful walking, meditation and contemplation are all well described methods for enhancing this awareness and mindfulness.

In summary, the compassionate activist recognizes that he/she too needs to be humanized and needs also to be liberated. The compassionate activist does not just regard the other person as in need of 'solution' or 'fixing'. They regard themselves as also warranting transformation in a process of care and compassion. This is perhaps their most distinctive feature and one I believe that is essential in order to achieve authentic integral social care and to ensure their own well-being in often difficult and challenging relationships.

Compassion

Compassion can be defined as an empathic response to the suffering or oppression of another and a desire to bring about their happiness and well-being through helping to end or mitigate that suffering. It is emphatically not pity nor should it be patronizing. It is grounded in empathy which is the capacity to understand and relate to the feelings and circumstances of another person. Empathy is rooted in the recognition in oneself of the feelings and experiences of the other person. Compassion also involves non-judgmental acceptance of the other. Acceptance is the necessary prerequisite for authentic relationships. In order to initiate effective and authentic relationships it is crucial to escape the limits of the judging mind.

> The beginning of compassion both to oneself and to others is in decreasing the number of judgements. I begin to see what is there without continuously labeling the events with the colours of my judgements and values. (Brandon 1976: 48)

As has been argued above, the first step in cultivating compassion is self-knowledge and self-care. We must acknowledge our own human frailty and dignity and that in each of us is the longing for liberation. Knowing where and how we suffer allows us to recognize the exact same sufferings and desires in others, even if, on occasion, the scale is quite different. In this way, compassion moves us beyond the categories of 'me and you' and of 'us and them' and leads us instead to the recognition that there is really only 'we together'. Thus, the second step in cultivating compassion is to recognize the humanity of the other. We must, as suggested above, meet the other on the plain of our common humanity.

Indeed, our own individual sufferings may actually prove to be our greatest teachers. Suffering can break the hold over us of certain illusions such as that we are different from everyone else, that we are self-reliant and independent of others or that we are in full control over our lives and need no one else. If we respond to our own suffering with openness and acceptance then it can lead almost inevitably to recognize and empathize with the suffering of others. Acknowledging our own vulnerabilities allows us to let go our temptation to power and to claim expertise over others. Ultimately, we are simply human beings together, united by our common sufferings and desires and capable of being bound together in mutual care for each other.

While we may not be able to ultimately liberate others from their various oppressions, compassion at the very least should be manifested in not doing harm to others. Integral social care should have 'non-harm' as a fundamental ethical principle. This ethic can be manifested in both words and actions. We must say or do nothing that would add to the oppression of another and that would in any way diminish their humanity. We must do nothing that would cause the other suffering.

Here indeed is a universally available ethic of care. The principle of non-harm can be found across all religions, secular systems of morals and cultures. It is an easily understood practice while, of course, difficult to actually observe in every situation. Embedded as we are within highly complex and interdependent social worlds, we do harm continually by virtue of our socio-structural order. Inequality, pollution, unfair trade and exploitation are endemic features of our social world. Simply by being part of this social world we are implicated in all of these. But this does not mean that non-harm cannot be a practice that we can begin within our interpersonal networks and seek to extend outwards in a committed compassionate activism. Doing no-harm is a simple, modest, unpretentious ethic yet one profoundly challenging and transformative at a personal and socio-political level.

If we truly observe the social world about us, both nationally and globally, we cannot fail to see the overwhelming reality of the poor, the excluded and the oppressed. The world of oppression is a fact and with that fact comes the response of compassion which is the yearning to bring about liberation. Hence, the compassionate activist must understand the practice of care as encompassing their immediate interpersonal dimensions as well as the wider socio-political world.

This minimum compassionate ethic of non-harm impels us to avoid doing things which cause suffering or oppression. We have a choice – either to add to the sum of suffering or to add to the sum of compassion. Each word and action of ours inevitably can do one or other. In our attitudes, our caring and our consuming we are faced with this choice. In this way, the compassionate activist has the potential to create the world anew. Either they can reproduce the world of oppression or they can transform it to a world of liberation.

At the end of the day, it may well be that there is no ultimate self-evident basis to choose one over the other. Indeed, there are many apparently compelling reasons and advantages in looking after oneself first and foremost. As we have consistently conceded, the claim that compassion is the gateway to humanization and happiness may only be 'proven' through direct experience rather than convincing argument. You have to just live it and see what happens. However, because care and compassion are so fundamental to our humanity, I am tempted to assert that because we *can* practise and cultivate more of this then we *ought* to. We can decide in a sense to humanize ourselves. We can choose better versions of ourselves. We can choose to forge better visions of ourselves and of our shared social and ecological worlds.

Boundaries

Of course, there are limits to care. We can after all only do so much. We cannot address and attend to every problem. At its most basic, the 'economy of love' means that we have to prioritize and compartmentalize our care practice. For example, it would not be reasonable to neglect one's own dependent infant in favour of a person who one has just encountered in the street. There is a rational order to how we manifest care. We simply cannot give equal care to each person that we encounter.

Boundaries refer to the setting of limits in our care relationships. They refer to our recognition of what we cannot do and what we should not do in those relationships. Many of these boundary limits have been discussed above. Important maxims were outlined such as 'I must be clear what my role is'; 'I am not the other'; I am not responsible for the other's service outcome'; 'I am responsible for a caring, compassionate and competent process'; 'I am not my job'.

In professional practice, boundaries are defined and set by the organization and sometimes by law. Organizational boundaries are contained in various policies, procedures and protocols and are implicit in the organization's values. But boundaries must also be set by the integral social carer themselves. These boundaries centre on how the carer determines the balance between the personal self and the professional self, or between home and work.

Boundaries are hugely important in defining the limits and scope of the relationship. As has been noted above, boundaries are not uniquely a feature of social care relationships. Boundaries occur in all relationships and are necessary in order to make them secure and safe. It is part of appropriate social behaviour to know and observe these boundaries.

Of course, social care relationships carry specific dangers regarding power imbalances and vulnerabilities. Therefore, understanding and observing boundaries take on even greater importance. One key boundary which was emphasized above is that the professional carer should never use the service user for their own needs or purposes. As was suggested, this may occur in quite subtle ways such as needing the suffering of the other person in order to validate one's own value. It is precisely to avoid these abuses that we have placed such emphasis on the notion of authenticity. The integral carer must be authentic in all of the senses described by Rogers. The authentic practitioner therefore should be one capable of vigilance and reflection and continually posing to himself/herself the questions designed to ensure boundary maintenance:

Whose needs are being met or coming first in this relationship?
What is appropriate for me to do given my current training and role?
What parts of my personal self is appropriate to disclose and share?
What are my personal and the organization's values?
When do I say 'no' in the work I undertake?

Saying no – in effect, putting a limit on the relationship – is the key, critical moment defining that relationship. Often, we are afraid to say no because we fear that the other person will as a result reject us. We may have become dependent on their affirmation of us and fear the loss of their regard. However, saying no is an inherent part of any relationship and, if that relationship is properly grounded in non-judgemental acceptance, should not undermine the basic security and continuity of the relationship. Indeed, it may only be at this point that the relationship may develop into something deeper and more real.

Finally, however, boundaries should not be turned into barriers designed to repel or reject the other person. Boundaries should be rooted in compassion and designed to facilitate an authentic and liberating relationship. We should not hide behind them or erect them as obstacles shielding us from the other person. One particular risk is that the carer subsumes himself/herself into his/her organizational role and becomes in effect an organizational cipher. In this case, they may lose their individuality and unique personhood and become merely the human mask of an impersonal corporate entity. Too many people fall into this trap, one that effectively hands over their moral autonomy to the organization. We in Ireland have seen this graphically illustrated once again in the Ryan and Murphy reports which showed that, despite extraordinary and appalling levels of institutional abuse, almost nobody in the religious and Catholic Church structures ever dissented publicly over a period of decades. This amounts to a comprehensive moral indictment of those bodies. The lesson is clear. The integral carer should never hide behind institutional boundaries if this involves the dehumanization of another. At the risk of repetition – the carer's moral autonomy should never be abandoned, even to an institution purportedly intended to do good.

Communication

Communication is often posited as the key skill required for the professional social carer. It is assumed that the quality of the care relationships is determined by the quality of the communication. However, communication is frequently presented as primarily involving a set of *techniques* which can be learned. Hence, the plethora of communications courses and aids now offered to professionals in pretty much every possible field.

The truth is however that genuine communication is not simply about the transmission of information or data from a source to a receiver. It is rather an aspect of the very complex dynamics involved in an interpersonal relationship. Communication involves a highly sophisticated social and cultural exchange and is accordingly affected by a variety of social factors such as social and linguistic conventions, emotional and intellectual experience, social position and relative power. Thus, it reflects and reinforces sociality and social roles.

In short, communication is about more than conveying information. It is primarily about achieving a *shared understanding* so that we gain appropriate insight and sensitivity to the perceptions and experiences of the other person. It is therefore necessarily a socio-cultural process. Achieving a shared understanding involves us in entering empathically into the other person's frames of reference and requires us to listen with understanding in a process of open dialogue involving word and response.

For Rogers the barrier to interpersonal, effective communication is that we do not really listen to the other person. We fail to truly listen because of our tendency to judge, evaluate and approve or disapprove of the other. To listen with understanding is to try and see from the other person's point of view and to suspend our evaluative reflexes. It is difficult to do this because it may take courage on our part due to the possibility that, if we really engage with the other person, we may find that he or she reveals something new to us about ourselves or the world and that as a result we may have to change. It is also difficult to do because it may involve us having to overcome, or set aside, our emotional responses to the other person such as anger, rejection or indifference, the very emotions which are preventing us listening to him/her in the first place.

Rogers suggests a method whereby one is obliged, before speaking oneself, to repeat back to the speaker what he/she has just said and, only if he/she agrees that you have truly expressed their view, then you may speak. This simple but difficult technique is designed to ensure effective listening particularly in situations of conflict.

We can therefore see that genuine communication is embedded into the dynamics of authentic relationships. The primary attribute of effective communication is to listen. We should listen with understanding by trying to grasp exactly what the other person is attempting to convey. As part of this, we should *listen with our eyes* in order to see the body language and physical demeanour of the other. As is well known, communication occurs through the body – the face, eyes, posture, gestures – at far profounder levels than through words. Our words can say one thing but our bodies another. We can mask our words but it is far more difficult to mask our bodies. Hence, the integral carer should listen with their eyes and be attentive to the total physical presentation of the other person. Once we realize that all behaviour is communication we understand that we must attend to all aspects of the appearance of the person before us.

Older, classical depictions of communication may in fact prove to be far more valuable and helpful than many modern ones. Aristotelian rhetoric for example describes communication as a social process which involves bringing home to the mind of the listener what it is that the speaker wishes to convey.[3] This conveying of meaning may well be enhanced by certain communicative technical skills but far more than that it requires a cultural and psychological understanding of one's interlocutor. Aristotle conceives of communication or argument as involving an interpersonal exchange encompassing ethos, pathos and logos.

Ethos refers to the personal character of the speaker. Do they have a sound grasp of practical reasoning? Have they a human or moral fitness for dealing with the matter under consideration? Finally, do they convey that they are well-disposed towards their interlocutor/s? Clearly, the personal character of the speaker is of great importance in determining the quality and authenticity of their communication. We judge the truth and value of verbal and communicative content all the time by who the person is who speaks. Thus, discredited persons or organizations undermine the truth content of their communication irrespective of the technical quality of that message. Credibility and trustworthiness, once lost, is gone almost forever. The integral social carer needs to pay close attention to this observation.

Pathos refers to the capacity of the speaker to put his/her interlocutor/s into a certain receptive frame of mind. This implies that the speaker understands the social and psychological context of the communication. He/she must show empathy and compassion in order to evoke or encourage openness to his/her argument on the part of his/her listener. In short, he/she must know when and how to speak and convey his/her message in order to maximize the chances that it will be received as he/she intended it. Finally, he/she must be aware of, and pay attention to, the various non-cognitive dimensions of the communication. This may involve its physical setting, environmental factors and various distractions.

---

3   For a modern, applied treatment of rhetoric see the outstanding work of Ricca Edmondson, particularly her book *Rhetoric in Sociology* (1984, Salem, MA: Salem House Academic Division) and her chapter 'Intercultural Rhetoric, Environmental Reasoning and Wise Argument' in R. Edmondson and H. Rau (eds) (2008), *Environmental Argument and Cultural Difference – Locations, Fractures and Deliberations*, Bern: Peter Lang AG. I am indebted to her for an appreciation of the contemporary value of classical rhetoric.

Finally, logos refers to the abstract, intellectual structure of what is to be communicated. What words to use, in what order and with what emphasis are all aspects of this consideration.

This analysis alerts us to the interpersonal and intercultural complexity of the communication process and that far more than simply using the right words is involved. Authenticity is in fact the key to effective communication. The more authentic and congruent the speaker, the more his/her words ring true and are likely to be received by the listener. Furthermore, the more authentic the speaker the more likely they are to be attentive to the listener. Thus, authenticity becomes the prerequisite for effective communication in the exact same manner in which it is the prerequisite for a real and liberating relationship.

In Chapter Eight we will emphasize the central importance of dialogue as a methodology for integral social care practice. Dialogue refers to both listening and responding to the person who speaks. However, as we shall see, dialogue is not simply a *tool* for relating to people. Dialogue constitutes our very humanity. As the philosopher Mikhail Bakhtin has eloquently put it:

> authentic human life is the open-ended dialogue. Life by its very nature is dialogic. To live means to participate in dialogue: to ask questions, to heed, to respond, to agree, and so forth. In this dialogue a person participates wholly and throughout his whole life: with his eyes, lips, hands, soul, spirit, with his whole body and deeds. He invests his entire self in discourse, and this discourse enters into the dialogic fabric of human life, into the world symposium. (Bakhtin 1984: 293)

Finally, communication in the socio-political sphere is affected by various cultural, institutional and ideological constraints. These constraints may give rise to a 'culture of silence' by which certain actors and certain political views and discourses are effectively removed from public articulation. As noted above, a key reason for this is the dominance in public discourse of a certain version of economic rationality. Anyone attempting to speak outside the categories of that discourse can be labeled and dismissed as 'irrational'. The effect of this is to close down the capacity to speak in terms other than those of the dominant discourse. How then can you put into words your concerns and demands where the words available to you are limited by various discursive constraints and by criteria of convention and relevance? How do you risk trying to break out of these limits when to do so may lead you open to charges of irrationality and non-sense and hence, leave you more likely to be defeated, or ignored, in public debate? Marcuse's nightmare that reason has come to identify itself with reality has come to pass.[4]

The result is that much that is important – even crucial to our humanity and understanding of our humanity – does not get heard in the formal public sphere. The consequence is that we do not gain a sense of what is being truly argued about, what is really at stake in contemporary politics and campaigns. Thus, we often do not have to address fundamental questions and challenges and we certainly rarely engage in a politics that is obliged to consider what is the 'good life' and what it is to be fully human.

We need to recognize that public debate is not like a discussion between two people. Indeed, thinking that it is offers a good example of how easily we are misled by false metaphors. The false analogy of two speakers suggests that each one knows their own position, has clear and understandable points to make, is willing to argue and to listen, is dialoguing as a relative equal and has the capacity to change their own and the other's mind. Our public debates are nothing like that.

Instead, campaigns, social movements, civil society actors of all kinds, and compassionate activists are battling not just entrenched forms of power held by particular actors, they are also battling convention, 'normality', 'common sense' and the various constructed forms of rationality. They are attempting to make new claims, new ways of seeing the world. But because this involves new language this is particularly challenging. This is because our language is ensnared in contemporary cultural practices and assumptions that are forcing us to see the world in a particular way. We certainly need a new language of politics, one that can celebrate and articulate integral social care and compassion.

---

4   For an interesting contemporary treatment of this issue see the work of Jean Rancière, for example *Disagreement: Politics and Philosophy* (1998, University of Minnesota Press).

Much that is important – even crucial to our humanity and understanding of our humanity – does not get heard in the formal public sphere.
Those who are oppressed are rarely heard and, when they do speak, are often
forced to use the dominant language and concepts that are culturally and
institutionally available. The result is that we do not gain a sense of what
is truly going on and what is truly important.

This in turn has serious implications for those trying to achieve social
and political change. If imagination is limited by what is expressible then
we are losing in our public discourse vast realms of what is possible.

Ethics

Ethical competence is a matter of such importance that it will be addressed
specifically in Chapter Nine below. Much has already been said in this
book about ethics to demonstrate that this is not an optional extra that the
integral social carer should take into account. The contrary is the case. An
ethical commitment is fundamental to integral social care practice. This
is because we are dealing with human beings and there is no more serious
and profound interaction possible. Social care ethics are grounded in the
recognition of the intrinsic value of each person irrespective of their utility or economic function. Simply by being alive, each person is of inherent
and inalienable value. Any harm done to that person or any rendering of
them into an object is ethically unacceptable.

All professional social care in Ireland operates in the dark and appalling shadow of the Ryan and Murphy reports. We have had occasion to
refer to these reports a number of times already. The *Ryan Report* in particular showed that an entire institutional framework of care, lasting for
many decades, was actually a system of abuse. Scores, probably hundreds,
of carers participated in sexual, emotional and physical abuse of vulnerable young people. Almost no one in the system dissented publicly. How

could this have happened?[5] One answer lies in the dreadful combination of power and ideology which gave Catholic Church agents social sanction to do as they wished with impunity. But another answer must point to a profound ethical failure, a profound failure to respect the intrinsic value of each person. There is a brutal irony in this given that we are speaking about an institution ostensibly grounded on a moral and religious worldview. It is clear that one over-riding lesson that we must learn is that when the first principles of person-centred ethics are abandoned then everything becomes possible.

The story of the institutions of care – whether it be the reformatory schools, the Borstals, the Magdalene laundries, the residential homes for young and old, the prisons, the psychiatric hospitals, the direct provision hostels – is that an ethical framework must be central and genuinely at the heart of what care practice is. In the face of the logic and modes of operation of all institutional systems we must always err on the side of humanity and never participate in causing harm to another.

Knowledge

The integral social carer must have specific knowledge. It is not enough to be well-meaning and well-disposed. They are also required to be effective. This means gaining access to particular bodies of knowledge in the social sciences, especially sociology, political science, philosophy and psychology. Also, the integral carer should benefit from the insights of various spiritual disciplines, anthropology and various applied subjects such as advocacy, human rights and ecology. All of this is simply to ensure that the integral carer has as rounded and comprehensive an understanding as possible

---

5   For a deeper treatment of this specific issue see Amnesty International's *In Plain Sight* report (2011).

about the subject of their care relationships – the human person in their full interpersonal and socio-political dimensions.

One aspect of the move towards professionalization is the consequent claim that social care makes to possess a specialized body of knowledge. In truth, I suspect that integral social care is as yet under-theorized and operates with a whole series of assumptions that, as of yet, have not been rigorously questioned. This book is merely one contribution to a critical reflection on the meaning of integral care in twenty-first-century capitalist societies. There are and, hopefully, will be others.

Of importance in developing its knowledge and understanding is that integral social care needs to continue to move away from a quasi-medical framework by which care work is often seen as an adjunct to health support and a version of health promotion. The fact is that the 'medicalization' of social issues and problems is more of an impediment to a proper response to personal and social challenges than an aid. Charitable and paternalistic conceptions of care also need to be finally and firmly let go.

In place of these older frameworks of understanding, the argument of this book has been that integral social care involves a compassionate response to the oppression of human beings that encompasses both inter-personal and socio-political dimensions. For this reason, the integral carer requires knowledge in each sphere in order that he/she may engage effectively for the integral liberation of all. This therefore is a radical reconceptualization of integral care best captured, we have proposed, by regarding such care practice as compassionate activism.

Technical skills

Finally, the social carer requires a series of more technical skills and competencies. This should at least include non-violent crisis intervention training; communication skills (within the framework outlined above); human rights; advocacy; dialogic practice; and inter-cultural training. This is not an exhaustive list by any means. As we will examine in greater detail in Parts Three and Four, the integral social carer should be someone dedicated to achieving human liberation and should be an agent of integral social change.

There is no pretence to neutrality here. The compassionate activist should be clearly committed to those who are oppressed and, if they do not come from that world themselves, seek to see reality from their perspective. Their project is to enter the world of the oppressed through authentic and liberating relationships and, with them and on their behalf, engage in personal and political activism primarily centred on disseminating and creating knowledge and analysis in order to bring about social change. This involves a training in critical consciousness so that the ideological structure maintaining inequality can be exposed and contested.

In summary, the compassionate activist is someone who believes in humanity and the possibility that humanity can enhance its capacities and structures of care and compassion. The compassionate activist should know reality as it is and, in particular, they should know the world of the oppressed. Of course, many will be from that world themselves. As noted above, much care work is carried out in particular by women, in both formal and informal settings, who are themselves oppressed in many ways, not least in the low status and recognition often accorded to their work. The hope of all compassionate activists should therefore be for a world of solidarity and justice, where the basic needs of all are met. They should be able to relate authentically to those who are suffering oppression either due to personal or social causes and they should be able to work with others to create new alternative models that can serve to humanize all aspects of society.

The next parts of this book address more comprehensively these more political and social aspects of integral social care. In doing so, we will rely initially on the ideas of Paulo Freire, particularly in so far as they serve as a foundation for developing our understanding of the centrality of dialogic practice.

PART THREE

The Socio-Political Dimension

CHAPTER SIX

Paulo Freire:
A Framework for Social and Political Liberation

Integral social care is care for the whole person. This means that the person is conceptualized in both their interpersonal and socio-political dimensions. For this reason, integral care can be distinguished from more traditional formulations of care practices which placed greater focus on the more immediate and personal aspects of the individual's needs and concerns. Hence, the sites where traditional care was practised were likely to be institutions, clinics, residential units and respite homes. The sites of integral care practice extend into domestic homes, communities, the media and politics. Integral care recognizes that the person and their social status are the product of various complex social and cultural forces. The individual person's total existential situation is not simply due to their personal choices and capabilities. It is therefore not solely their responsibility. Because their situation is also the result of social and political factors and options it is also the responsibility of all of us. Thus, the status and life opportunities of people with disabilities, or of Travellers, or of homeless people, or of ethnic minorities and so on reflect not just the turning points and crisis moments of their personal biographies but it also reflects the wider values and choices of our society as determined politically.

Yet, despite over a century of social science study, many people still find it difficult to recognize the individual person as the product of both personal and social factors. Thus, a criminal remains someone who is widely regarded as entirely and individually responsible for their criminality. Their social circumstances, their socialization, their economic and educational constraints and their limited opportunities generally, while acknowledged to be of some impact, are not popularly regarded as sufficient to explain or account for their behaviour. (Justifying it is of course a different issue). In part, as we have suggested in previous chapters, this understanding is the result of a powerful ideological construction which posits the self-interested rational individual as the true description of the human person. In similar vein, we may still think of the social world as a 'natural', unquestionable fixed entity which is set up as it is due to some inevitable process derived from human nature and from inexorable rules of sociality and behaviour. This essentialist conception of the person and of society leads many to conclude that the world simply is as it must be and cannot be other. Within this perspective we may well regret aspects of it but take the view that there is nothing that we can do. This is how the world is. It is as though society has dropped from the heavens fully formed, with people already in it, and we can do little about it.

As we have argued above, this perspective suffers from a fundamental misunderstanding of social structure and how social structure influences and constructs social behaviour and relations. Perhaps the most helpful analyst who addresses how we might begin a process of critical under-standing of our social reality is the Brazilian educationalist Paulo Freire. The ideas of Freire run counter to many of the dominant discourses and ideologies that have shaped Western politics particularly in the last three decades. Whether we designate these dominant discourses as neo-liberalism or neo-conservatism or free-market fundamentalism, one of the aspects of their dominance is that they inculcate a sense of fatalism. This is because they appear so powerful and so entrenched that there appears no alterna-tive to the economic, political and social system that they describe and consequently also no way of resisting them. In addition, because they claim that the social world as constructed by them is in fact 'natural' and based on fundamental laws of human and social nature, there appears to be liter-ally no point in resisting them. The society they have forged is regarded as inevitable and inexorable. The claim made is that there simply is no possible workable alternative that could be better in tune with human nature.

Much of Freire's work can be understood as an attempt to overcome this induced systemic fatalism. Instead, Freire placed key emphasis on the need to forge a critical consciousness so that the oppressive or inhibiting social realities confronting people can be directly and effectively challenged and changed. In a word, he re-affirmed the empirical reality that the world can be understood as constructed and consequently it can be changed. It is with this emphasis on the possibility of progressive and humanizing change that Freire's work offers particular advantages and insights to the integral social carer.

Of course, as the well known Freirean scholar Peter Mayo[1] notes, 'The greatest and most enduring aspect of Freire's work is his emphasis on the political nature of all educational activity' (Mayo 2009: 2). As we have similarly suggested in regards to social care practice, education either domesticates or liberates. For Freire, emancipatory education through dialogue is the key tool for developing critical awareness and empowering people to change social reality itself.

But 'education' is not just something that happens in formally recognized institutions of learning. Adult pedagogy occurs in multiple settings and sites and thus is not so much a public good to be produced and consumed but rather is an instrument and methodology of liberation and humanization to be disseminated throughout society. In this sense, the integral social carer can be thought of also to be an adult pedagogical worker who is seeking to achieve with others through his/her social care relationships a new, critical understanding of the world, precisely in order that that world can be changed.

Achieving humanization is perhaps the whole goal of Freire's concerns. It is specifically in this commitment to humanization that Freire's work has compelling appeal and importance to any rigorous exploration of integral social care. His insistence that genuine conscientization and democratization leads to a personal and social transformation towards greater humanization reminds us that being fully human is ultimately the goal and final measure for any 'social care' worthy of the name. It also reminds us that integral social care should always be developmental and transformative. In so far as it is, then social care is a project of hope – hope that a better world is possible and attainable.

1 See for example P. Mayo (2009), *Liberating Praxis – Paulo Freire's Legacy for Radical Education and Politics*, Rotterdam: Sense Publishers.

Freire's *Pedagogy of the Oppressed*

Freire's best known and most influential text is *Pedagogy of the Oppressed*.[2] The book was written while he was in exile in Chile following the Brazilian military coup of 1964. Published in 1970, it was based on many years of direct experience of working with the poor of Brazil and Chile. Perhaps as many as 80 per cent of the population of South America were living at the time in conditions of dire poverty.

Freire was born in 1921 in Recife, Brazil. While initially he taught Portuguese in secondary schools, from 1946 he began developing adult literacy programmes. That work was brought to an end with the military coup. Following a brief imprisonment he went into exile in Chile. After the Portuguese language publication of *Pedagogy of the Oppressed* he was invited in 1969 to Harvard as a visiting Professor. He later moved to Europe as a special education advisor to the World Council of Churches. He finally returned to Brazil in 1980 where he took up again his work in adult pedagogy. He was appointed in 1988 as Secretary of Education in Sao Paulo by the Brazilian Workers Party. Freire died in 1997.

As we shall discuss in the next chapter, we still live in a world marred by widespread and systematic poverty. Added to the threats posed by war and nuclear proliferation is the realization that the planet's ecology is in crisis as a consequence of human action. In this context, Freire's work offers us enduring and significant ideas regarding the importance of developing a critical consciousness; the necessity of affirming the project of humanization; and the centrality and necessity of dialogue as the key tool for social progress. It seems to me that these are three values of the utmost importance for compassionate activism, values which can act as an essential tool to assess the competing political ideologies confronting us today. Freire opposed all

---

2   Much of this chapter is drawn directly from my chapter 'Opening up Paulo Freire's Pedagogy of the Oppressed', in Fiona Dukelow and Orla O Donovan (eds) (2010), *Opening up Classic Texts*, Manchester: Manchester University Press.

received and dogmatic versions of social reality, from both left and right – 'They both suffer from an absence of doubt' (Freire 1972: 18).[3]

In fact, *Pedagogy of the Oppressed* is a ringing invocation of the necessity (both empirical and normative) for human freedom. Throughout the text, Freire contrasts oppression and liberation. These are the two polarities of the human existential condition. On the one hand, the poor are oppressed by virtue of their poverty and are unable to be themselves as free, human subjects. Yet they may accept this situation as fated or unalterable. They may even fear freedom because it carries risk and the potential for conflict. In addition, in situations of objective oppression and mass poverty, the rich are not free either. They too live in fear and destroy their own humanity by their violent suppression of their fellow human beings. Freire's book can be understood as providing a method to enable the poor to understand the structural reasons for their poverty so that they can begin to liberate themselves and become free, autonomous human beings. By so doing they liberate their oppressors too.

The key tool identified by Freire for achieving this liberation is education. Freire argues for a new type of education – an education or pedagogy *of* the oppressed, i.e. one constructed by themselves, out of their lived experience. Conventional education is critiqued by Freire as embedded within oppressive structures. Such education is designed to pacify, to render the student a compliant object to be controlled. To overcome this reality, Freire develops a number of key concepts – problematization, de-mythologization, conscientization, the culture of silence. It's here above all else I think that we might find Freire's contemporary relevance and enduring inspiration for compassionate activism. Our education and ideological system remains co-opted into an economic imperative centred on growth and inequality. Certain voices and certain words are today reduced to silence in the public sphere. How to speak straightforwardly out of one's direct experience remains problematic. As we have noted above, oppressed groups are obliged

---

3   The page numbers cited are from Paulo Freire (1972), *Pedagogy of the Oppressed*, London: Penguin Books. Note that throughout Freire uses gendered terminology when referring to human beings.

to translate their concerns into other language, especially the language of
economics and business. Even the term 'the oppressed' is politically potent
and almost never used to designate an empirically identifiable group of
people. Thus, officially, we don't have 'oppressed' in Ireland.

A key moment in the path of liberation is when the poor ask what is
the nature of the social world. Is it really like the 'natural' world, i.e. governed by laws and irrevocable processes? Or is it malleable – subject to
human agency – and capable of being constructed and re-constructed?
The realization that social reality is constructed and that we can understand how it is constructed and how it may be changed is the key moment
when one moves from a naïve, mythical view of the world to an analytical
understanding. Freire's normative or ethical claim is that the social world
should not have 'oppression', i.e. any curtailment of freedom. The goal of
a proper social system should be maximum humanization.

This vision of humanization both as the *end* of political activity and
as the criteria for determining the *means* by which political action is conducted seems to me particularly exciting and corresponds closely to how
we have described integral social care. Freire offers an approach which
combines political, philosophical and cultural methods to achieve radical
social change but refuses to subordinate means to ends. The integral social
carer cannot fail to glimpse the value of Freire's emphasis on reading reality
'from below', i.e. from the perspective of the poor and oppressed, rather
than imposing theoretical frameworks of liberation or service delivery
on them. The intrinsic value of giving the poor and oppressed their own
voices and their own words, has I believe enormous modern potency and
value.[4] Indeed, Freire's work continues to implicitly challenge many of the
orthodoxies of contemporary social theory and social care practice.

Pedagogy of the Oppressed is a short book. Freire states that:

---

4   It should be noted once again that we are using the somewhat loaded term 'the poor'
     in this book to designate all of those suffering from social exclusion and marginali-
     zation, whether that is the result of economic, gender, ethnic, identity, biological or
     intellectual factors. Freire's early work may appear to have emphasized the materi-
     ally poor in particular but they were the overwhelming human reality that he was
     addressing.

This book will present some aspects of what the writer has termed the 'pedagogy of the oppressed', a pedagogy which must be forged *with*, not *for*, the oppressed (be they individuals or whole peoples) in the incessant struggle to regain their humanity. This pedagogy makes oppression and its causes objects of reflection by the oppressed, and from that reflection will come their necessary engagement in the struggle for their liberation. And in the struggle this pedagogy will be made and remade. (25)

Freedom

The core problematic addressed in the book's first chapter is what it is to be human. Key to this for Freire is freedom. Freedom is '... the indispensable condition for the quest for human completeness' (24). The struggle to be human begins in the struggle to be free. One can detect in Freire's work here a very strong influence from European existentialism, especially ideas developed by Sartre regarding how the human subject is made through one's actions and choices. However, in the Latin American situation, this question is posed in the context of empirical dehumanization through poverty. In every situation and conflict, the issue of humanization is always at stake. In claiming their humanity, the oppressed should not themselves become oppressors. This is a risk because initially, in liberating themselves, the oppressed are tempted to become like their oppressors because this is their model for what it is to be human and free.

Crucial to beginning the process of liberation is the awareness of oppression. Oppression is defined as:

Any situation in which A objectively exploits B or hinders his pursuit of self-affirmation as a responsible person is one of oppression. (31)

Oppression interferes with the person's ontological and historical vocation to be more fully human. Oppression is kept in place by fatalism – the belief that one's social condition is the result of destiny, fate, fortune, God's will, magic, or myth. Self-depreciation and feelings of worthlessness accentuate this passivity. What is required to overcome this is a new liberating praxis – 'reflection and action upon the world in order to transform it' (28). This can happen when people realize that it is we ourselves who produce our social reality. Thus we can change it.

The key to awakening awareness and liberation among the oppressed is critical and liberating dialogue. This is a point of the utmost importance for Freire. 'One must trust the oppressed and in their ability to reason' (41). Action must be based on pedagogy not propaganda. Simplistic programmes, slogans and deductive political templates are not of value. In fact, they can form part of the oppressive disempowerment of the people.

Pedagogy

In the second chapter Freire turns his attention specifically to the education system and models of pedagogy. He asserts that contemporary education has a narrative character – it suffers from 'narration sickness' (45).

> Narration (with the teacher as narrator) leads the students to memorize mechanically the narrated content. Worse still, it turns them into 'containers', into receptacles to be filled by the teacher. The more completely he fills the receptacles, the better a teacher he is. The more meekly the receptacles permit themselves to be filled, the better students they are. (45)

In this style of 'banking' education there is a focus on memory, repetition and rote learning. The objective is to turn people into automatons. 'The educated man is the adapted man, because he is "more fit" for the world' (50). For this reason, banking methods cannot be used for the purposes of liberation because its objective is to change the consciousness of the oppressed so they adapt to the situation of oppression.

The alternative to this is 'problem posing' education engaged in through dialogical relations. Dialogue is the critical method involving an engagement between student-teacher and teacher-student. The goal of liberatory education is the end of the teacher-student contradiction. The objective is to achieve critical cognition, where the students are 'critical co-investigators in dialogue with the teacher' (54). The consequence of 'problem-posing education' is men develop their power to perceive critically *the way they exist* in the world *with which* and *in which* they find themselves; they come to see the world not as a static reality, but as a reality in process, in transformation. (56)

Banking education mythicizes reality whereas problem-posing education de-mythologizes it. People come to realize that they can control social reality. In this context, the subversive power of the question 'why' is revealed – 'No oppressive order could permit the oppressed to begin to question: Why?' (59).

Dialogue

In Chapter Three Freire addresses his key concern with dialogue.

Dialogue is the encounter between men, mediated by the world, in order to name the world ... If it is in speaking their word that men transform the world by naming it, dialogue imposes itself as the way in which men achieve significance as men. Dialogue is thus an existential necessity. (61)

For Freire 'To speak a true word is to transform the world' (60). 'To exist, humanly, is to name the world, to change it' (61). For dialogue to be genuine and possible there must be love, faith, hope, humanity and trust. 'To glorify democracy and to silence the people is a farce; to discourse on humanism and to negate man is a lie' (64).

If I do not love the world – if I do not love life – if I do not love men – I cannot enter into dialogue. (62)

The objective of the pedagogy of liberation is now revealed as 'the dialogical man'. No libertarian programme can be imposed – that would simply be a return to a banking methodology. Instead, freedom is to be uncovered through the process of dialogue and engagement with the people. Any failure to respect the view of the world held by the people is 'cultural invasion', a point which he further develops in the fourth chapter.

The purpose of this process is to allow one to see critically. 'Conscientization is the deepening of the attitude of awareness characteristic of all emergence' (81). This method puts the student at the centre of the process.

Social change

Finally Freire outlines how radical social change can occur in situations of deep oppression. His concern however is to outline a process not a programme. Radical social change, he asserts throughout, can only emerge from dialogue with the people. 'Dialogue is a fundamental precondition for their true humanization' (107). The characteristics of anti-dialogical action carried out either by the oppressors or by would-be saviours of the people include:

- Conquest (a key method of which is by inculcating myths)
- Divide and rule (which includes not just dividing the people but also dividing up social problems and social perspectives by not seeing the connections between issues)
- Manipulation (one component of which is the false image of the people inculcated in them from the oppressors)
- Cultural invasion (by which the invaders 'impose their own view of the world upon those they invade and inhibit the creativity of the invaded by curbing their expression' (121))

By contrast, dialogical action – the object of which is to get the oppressed to transform unjust reality – is characterized by:

- Co-operation – 'subjects meet in cooperation in order to transform the world' (135)
- Unity for liberation
- Organization
- Cultural synthesis

Application to integral social care

Whereas Rogers' contribution to social care theory and practice is widely recognized, Freire's direct relevance may not seem as clear cut. Therefore, it is important, in the spirit of Freire's work itself, to subject this account to an initial critique. On the positive side, Freire confronts two domi-nant myths still prevalent in contemporary Western society and which we have made reference to on a number of occasions. First, is the myth of the individual as a kind of free-floating asocial being and second, that of the social world as static and 'natural', in the sense that its present form is inevitable and obvious. These myths taken together amount to a powerful ideological justification for a view of the world that posits personal effort and endeavour as the key criteria for achieving material and social success within a fixed and naturally constrained social world. The implication of this is that the poor are poor because of personal failure on their part and the rich are so because of personal virtues and talents. This view of the world, if internalized by the poor, can become a key component of the passivity, fatalism and low self-value which Freire identifies as inimical to their capacity to understand and change the world. Integral social care cannot fail to contest this false worldview.

However, there may also be a number of reasonable objections to the universal reach of Freire's arguments that warrant acknowledgement. The first might be to enquire whether, in the context particularly of European social democracy, the categories of oppressed and oppressor are so clear. Might there be a false dichotomization here not readily applicable outside of the poor Southern nations of the world? As noted above, there is a wider recognition today of the multiple forms that oppression takes which tran-scend material factors to include identity, gender, ethnicity, able-bodiness and so on.[5] In this context the only options may not be between oppression

5   See here the important work of Nancy Fraser (e.g. *Justice Interruptus – Critical Reflections on the 'Postsocialist' Condition*, 1997) in arguing for the need to identify a politics of social recognition as being as significant in modern societies as the more

and revolution. A middle-way may be possible. In addition, what happens if the people do not want revolution but reform? Will this be dismissed as evidence of false consciousness on their part?

A second issue that may be raised is whether the 'new person' heralded and lauded by Freire is possible outside of a religious or ethical framework? The invocation to faith, hope and love made by Freire clearly ring of Christian moral virtues rather than of a proletarian class consciousness. Once again, the foundation of these ideas within a specifically Christian Latin America may hinder their easy translation or application to societies whose religious and cultural ethos is non-Christian or even non-religious. In addition, Freire may be accused of being utopian in this regard. Will human beings really behave in this virtuous manner once material deprivation has been overcome?

Finally, one may also question whether Freire's pedagogical ideas themselves can have universal application. Is his depiction of 'banking' education a fair characterization of contemporary pedagogical practice? New educational theories now animate and inform practice in the Western world. In addition, a teaching methodology of teacher-student dialogue may not always be appropriate for every academic discipline and setting. One thinks of mathematics for example or many of the natural sciences. In these instances the teacher is required to be didactic in order to equip the student to understand and operationalize core concepts and tools. It may not be fair to characterize such pedagogy as necessarily oppressive.

Leaving aside these particular objections or cautions, the issue for us is how relevant is this Freirean perspective to integral social care? To pose this question slightly differently, what can integral social care find of value in Freire's ideas and concepts? An initial answer might begin empirically. Throughout the Southern world, and by no means limited to South America, Freirean approaches have had a significant and transforming impact. They have been tested and applied in a multitude of countries and

traditional politics of redistribution. She argues that social justice is not just about a distribution of resources but also requires the recognition of the equal status of diverse social actors as peer participants in the social world.

social circumstances. That Freirean ideas remain vibrant and in widespread use today can only testify to their validity and utility, particularly in situations of objective oppression. Freire's core ideas also remain unsettling and challenging to those who seek to uphold and defend the *status quo*.

In Ireland too, Freire's methodologies have shown themselves to have value and relevance. One of the most notable applications occurred in January 1985 when the returned Columban missionary John O'Connell established an educational programme with twenty four Traveller activists in Dublin. O'Connell had worked in the Philippines and was anxious to apply Freire's pedagogical ideas in Ireland. With others he established the Dublin Traveller Education and Training Group in 1985[6] and set out to create Freirean-based consciousness awareness groups. These were hugely successful and had a major impact on Traveller understanding of their social position and oppression in Irish society. It is clear that this early Freirean programme was a decisive moment in creating the modern Traveller rights movement.[7] Until this time, Travellers were largely characterized by attitudes of fatalism regarding their position, invoking 'God's will' as an explanatory framework for their disadvantage. The immediate effect of the programme was to change this language. From then on, Traveller activists spoke of oppression and characterized their campaigning as a struggle for liberation. As Martin Collins said when addressing the opening session of the National Seminar of Traveller Parents and Learners:

> Education needs to be about liberating Travellers, not about domesticating them. True Education will give Travellers the tools to challenge their oppression rather than teaching them how to become acceptable in a settled world.

Freirean pedagogy has also been used in adult education programmes throughout Ireland, particularly those aimed at disadvantaged and marginalized groups. Freire's influence can be seen for example in the founding of

---

6   In 1995 this became Pavee Point.
7   Michael Collins' wonderful one-person play *It's a cultural thing, or is it?* captures the immense impact of this programme on his and other young Travellers' understanding of their lived reality. As he says in the play – 'We learned the word discrimination.'

the Partners Training for Transformation, a series of development education programmes which began in 1981. This initiative, instigated both by people working in Ireland and returned development workers, set out to develop programmes for community education and empowerment focused on drawing from people's own experiences. Apart from their direct involvement in communities, the training manuals developed by the Partners further transmitted Freirean ideas in Ireland.

Thus, the value and utility of Freire's ideas have been clearly demonstrated. Where Rogers provides us with a helpful account of what it is to be a person, the great virtue of Freire's ideas for integral social care practice lies in their contribution to addressing two questions of the utmost importance which we have posed right at the outset of this book: what it is that we want to achieve in care and how do we get there. Freire offers us I believe profound answers to both of these questions. First, he presents humanization as the goal and purpose of any activism committed to freedom and well-being and, second, he offers us a humanized and humanizing methodology for achieving this. By adapting and applying these ideas to our care practice, we can receive two inestimable contributions to a re-invigorated theory of integral social care, one which can contribute significantly to bringing about a renewed vision and dignity to social care practice, a renewal which is sorely needed. Let us briefly take each question in turn.

First, what do we want to achieve? What is the purpose of our social care? This question has already been addressed in Chapter Four above. Freire's approach, as is Rogers', is firmly centred in humanist values that assert the freedom and dignity of the human person. The human person is realized through the free decisions he or she makes. Thus, the purpose and objective of Freire's pedagogy is bringing about humanization both for the individual and for the wider society. I have argued that that is precisely what integral social care should be about too. With this as our focus, we can then have the yardstick by which we can measure and determine our actions and strategies. We need to develop the conviction that what really matters in our practice is whether we are bringing about the humanization of each other or not.

Second, how do we get there? Freire's pedagogical method offers an empirically effective approach to working with people who are oppressed.

This involves a bottom-up practice in which dialogue and conscientization are central. In such an approach, the person himself, not an outside institution or an 'expert' who seeks to 'bank' answers or solutions, takes charge of their own supports and liberation. The person becomes the priority and leader of the process. The working methodology is one of open dialogue designed to develop the critical consciousness and awareness of the person, precisely so that they can liberate themselves from false and mythical understandings of themselves and of the wider social world. This will allow them exercise the maximum possible autonomy and choice. The process of dialogue is itself an integral part of humanization. Humanization cannot be delivered or banked as a product – it is formed through the process of open mutual dialogue through which the person is accepted and recognized as a subject, with their own view of the world and with their own choices to make freely. In Chapter Eight below I will build on this outline to suggest a specific methodology which seeks to further operationalize this approach.

Finally, Freire's work reminds us of two further fundamental facts which we have stressed throughout this book. First, a genuine human existence is characterized by freedom and solidarity. Both freedom and solidarity are needed in order to ensure a civilized, caring society. To bring this about, we need to recover the social efficacy and meaning of terms such as love, happiness, fraternity, care and compassion. These, after all, are the very constituents of human well-being and surely better describe a more inspiring vision of ourselves and our societies than concepts such as competition, efficiency, calculability, individualism and mutual forbearance.

Secondly, Freire also obliges us to recognize that the social world is not fixed or 'natural'. It is constructed by forces and structures which we can identify. As it is constructed so it can be reformed and changed and made subject to human agency. We can shape a social world as we wish and make it something that reflects and determines who we want to be. This is the utopian dream contained in a progressive and humanistic politics. Men and women discover in their actions on the social world that it can be re-formed and, in that very process itself, that they too can be humanized. What is of importance here is not that we have a pre-determined blueprint or master plan. No, the point is that if we proceed by a humanized process of democracy and dialogue, we will inevitably bring about the world we desire. This is a statement of hope and in this project the potential and nobility of a renewed compassionate social care activism can be located. Hope is essential in order to overcome our widespread passivity and fatalism. The next chapter seeks to further these reflections.

CHAPTER SEVEN

The Human Person as a Social Being

The human person is the subject and object of integral social care. Critically though, the human person is both an individual who is unique and valuable in themselves and also someone inexorably shaped and formed by wider socio-cultural forces. In classical sociology, this dual aspect of the person is often described as the agency-structure distinction. On the one hand, we know we exercise free choices and act in the social world in accordance with these (agency), yet we also know that how we choose, in what way we choose and what is available as choices are culturally and socially determined (structure). Where the balance lies between the two is the content of rich academic debate.

It is beyond the remit of this book to enter into this specific question. Instead, I want to more narrowly focus on the implications of this social scientific understanding of this dual aspect of the human being for our developing concept of integral social care. In doing so, we will move inevitably from the more secure ground of an empirical description of the social world into the more contentious and contestable ground of how we want the social world to be. Such a move, rooted within the tradition of critical social theory, draws its origins from Marx's famous Thesis 11 in *The Theses on Feuerbach*: 'Philosophers have hitherto only interpreted the world in various ways; the point is to change it.'

This question can be re-framed in another way, one that we have posed previously in this book. Given that the social world is constructed, and that human beings are in large part the products of that social world with their quality of life largely determined by their economic and social status, how then do we want that world to be? Crucial here is the recognition that it is we who make and shape that world. It is not a 'natural' entity over and above us. It is our creation.

When we look closely at the social world that we have created what do we see? This depends on our perspective, on our values and, perhaps most crucially of all, on our social position. How the social world appears to be depends on where we stand in that world. If we attempt an 'objective', empirical description we find that the social world presents many faces. On one side there is great material wealth and opulence and on the other great material poverty and deprivation. There is obesity and starvation. There are luxury villas and shantytowns. There are swimming pools and poisoned waterholes. For some, the existing state of affairs is hugely beneficial and brings about personal well-being. For others, the existing state of affairs is oppressive and results in suffering and deficiency. In short, for those who can readily access the resources created by our globalized world then that world appears to be a success. But for those who cannot access those resources, or not enough of those resources, then that world is a failure. The present structure of the world gives rise to a situation where there are those who gain, or who hope to gain, and there are those who must lose. As a result, there are those who wish to maintain the social world as it is and indeed extend its logic and there are those who wish to change it.

How are we to navigate our way through these competing claims and perspectives? Shying away from the challenge to do so is not a tenable option. Avoiding the arena of social conflict on the basis that we are doing the 'neutral' and unproblematic task of social care is at best disingenuous and at worst deliberate delusion. One's action in the social realm almost always either reproduces or transforms the existing social order, even in micro-minute ways. We are always choosing. The point is not to allow our choice be made by another, or by convention, or by forces greater than ourselves. The point is rather for ourselves to genuinely choose between reproducing the present state of affairs or transforming them.

The key criterion advanced by this book to guide us as social carers in making this choice is that integral social care practice is committed to achieving humanization, which is understood as a process of liberating the person from personal and social oppressions. For this reason, humanization is the supreme value which should underline all our practice. Based on that argument, I want to propose three propositions of liberation which will serve to guide how we might think about the meaning of freedom in the socio-political dimension. Following that, I will argue that the appropriate episte-mological perspective from which to view and judge social reality is that of the poor and oppressed as they can provide us with a genuinely empirical measure of the extent of our social care and compassion. In addition, I will attempt to show that how the social world is structured affects all of us, whether we are winners or losers. Finally, I will present five propositions which will attempt to provide a framework for integral social care practice in the socio-political dimension. In short, this chapter attempts to address the question as to what integral care should look like in the wider political realm.

The propositions of freedom

As these propositions are derived from the various arguments made above, they do not warrant further elaboration.

1. To be human is to be free.
    1.1 Any arbitrary curtailment of freedom is repressive.
    1.2 Repression is often experienced when you seek freedom.
    1.3 Freedom and humanization are the signs and goals of a civi-lized society.

2. To be human is to be social.
    2.1 The isolated subject is an illusion.
    2.2 We are responsible to, and for, each other.
    2.3 This implies solidarity.

3. The social world (history) can change and be more free and human.
    3.1 We are responsible for how the world is.
    3.2 Because we can re-fashion it we can create maximum libera-tion and social care.
    3.3 Competing social models of the world (politics) gives rise to conflict and potential oppression.

To summarize these propositions, we can say that human beings are free individuals, yet are social and therefore interdependent, and are capable of fashioning the social world in accordance with their values and visions. These are surely in themselves reasonable and uncontentious assertions which can be readily demonstrated historically. Much of the trajectory of modern Western history can be described as an unfolding process of liberation by which groups such as non-aristocrats, citizens, non-believers, women, blacks, homosexuals, and others finally attained recognition of their rights and identities. Nonetheless, it is important to observe that all of these extensions in social and political freedom necessitated conflict and persuasion and were more often than not met with initial opposition and repression. A simple history of the women's movement from the suffragettes on will clearly illustrate that.

Therefore, based on the historical record, it is likely that to any new claim to liberation or to any claim that society must change there will be resistance. As has been noted above, conflict is an inevitable feature of social groups, from the smallest to the biggest. In our highly complex modern social world, conflict and repression are no less a feature. Any action in the social world designed to change it will inevitably produce conflict. This conflict is often resolved not by force of argument or by considered and fair assessments of the legitimacy of the change being proposed but by the balance of power and resources between competing social actors. In this regard, the rich and powerful – those who benefit from the *status quo* – may be few in number but they are strong in power. By contrast, the poor and oppressed – those who suffer from the *status quo* – may be many in number but are weak in power. This is the political reality. Power in our globalized social world lies not solely in physical capability but far more importantly in the ability to control the symbolic and ideological structure by which the limits of the possible and the conceptual horizons of what constitutes the good life are set. Thus, certain proposals and certain demands can be dismissed by the simple judgement that they are not 'realistic'. The standards of what is 'realistic' and what 'living in the real world' entails are not, in fact, obvious. They are themselves socially constructed.

As we have suggested in Chapter Two above, our society is unprecedented in human cultural history by the deep penetration of social exhortations into our private life. The demands to consume, conveyed by an all pervasive media, saturate our radio, television, internet, streetscapes, magazines, sporting and cultural events, and so on. The act of consuming and the capacity to consume are presented before us as the epitome of rational behaviour and the marker of human success.

Yet, our consuming ties us structurally into a nexus of oppression and ecological destruction. It is for this reason that integral social care, which is so deeply rooted in our humanity, in order to be effective, must now, above all, become committed to social and structural transformation. Human compassion, grounded in the interpersonal, must become political to be fully efficacious. This is because our socio-political system is causing inherently good people (as almost all of us are) to do bad things. We therefore need to conceptualize our humanity – both who we are and what we are doing – in this wider structural dimension.

Seeing reality 'from below': an epistemological shift

One reasonably available way by which we can begin to see what we are doing is to shift our perspective on the world. If we could see reality from the perspective of those who are poor and oppressed (using these terms in the wide sense deployed in this book) – those in particular need of solidarity and care – then we would come to know the world in a new manner. We could see past the 'shadow world' of the wealthy and glamorous, the world which entrances us and offers us an idealization of our own aspirations. This world – the realm of celebrity and media – can give the appearance of substantiality in a culture such as our own where form often dominates over substance. Instead, if we look at the 'true world', where *most* people on our planet live, then we would see a world far from glamour and prosperity. The reason why seeing the social world 'from below' offers a better perspective is that, if we truly wish for humanization and liberation, then the existence of the poor and oppressed provides us with an objective measure of the extent of dehumanization that there actually is. The sheer empirical reality of the poor challenges our claims to be committed to human liberation. If we really care then, at first instance, we need to at least *see* the world of the poor.

In short, if we wish to correctly grasp the true reality of our social world then we need to see it 'from below', i.e. from the viewpoint of the poor. This involves coming to see the world from a new epistemological and methodological platform. Thus, in order to investigate the character of social reality, our new generating questions become what does this society or world look like from the position of the poor and how do we judge this society from their perspective. The poor can then become a measure of 'progress' and 'development' and can serve as the empirical judge of whether we have truly achieved humanization, freedom and justice for all. Their very reality (they are, after all, the global majority) can puncture the delusory bubble within which is contained our perceptions and illusions about what is really going on in our world.

Who, then, are the poor? The great El Salvadorian theologian Jon Sobrino has defined the global poor as those who do not take life for granted, as those who die before their time or as those who have nearly all the powers of the world against them, yet who still have an intrinsic humanizing power and potential which enables them to endure.[1] In more sociological terms, we might say that the poor are those who are denied or reduced as social beings, who are excluded from social fellowship or from freely and equally accessing the resources of their society. They are in this condition not primarily because of some personal flaw but because they have been deprived of social and political power by their low income, by their lack of employment, by their physical or intellectual disability, by their sickness or by their cultural status. The poor are not just those who are economically and materially disadvantaged. They are those whose status is reduced, whose identity is ignored, whose voices are silent, whose gender is considered inferior, whose nationality or ethnicity is suppressed or denied. In general terms, they are rendered poor (i.e. made impoverished) because

---

1   See Jon Sobrino (2008), *The Eye of the Needle – No Salvation outside the Poor, A Utopian-Prophetic Essay*, London: Dartman, Longman & Todd.

they have been excluded from material and symbolic resources and this exclusion, because it limits their freedom, amounts to objective oppression. Most, if not all, of those who seek professional social care come from this oppressed reality. As integral social carers, what is our response to be? Can it really be confined solely to the interpersonal dimension and ignore entirely the socio-political? Would that genuinely be integral care?

If the integral carer is to be intimately involved in the world of the poor, then surely, if they are not themselves directly from that world, they must come to know that world? If they are to non-judgementally accept the individuals who dwell there, then surely they must come to see through the eyes of that world? Surely, the appropriate authentic and epistemological perspective is that of the world of the poor? What is the world like from the viewpoint of those who are physically impaired, those who are in mental distress, those in material deprivation, those who are from excluded ethnic minorities? Drawing from the pedagogical methodology of Freire the first action of the critical educator is to know the social reality of those with whom we work. The alternative would be to view that world 'from above', that is to view it as an object needing 'normalization' and 'integration'. If we may be forgiven for referring to it one more time, the *Ryan Report* revealed to us in stark detail what care 'from above' can look like and what happens when the poor are rendered into objects deprived of autonomy and voice. Many, indeed most, of those incarcerated into Ireland's various institutions of care were economically and socially poor. In fact, many were incarcerated precisely *because* they were poor. There, they were subjected not to a process of liberation but one of further and deeper oppression.[2]

As we noted above, the specific additional value of this epistemological shift is that the existence of the poor provide us with a measure of 'progress' and 'development'. Their existence places our social world under judgement. Let us therefore quantify the reality of the poor and consider what the sheer scale and nature of this reality reveals about the character of our world.

2   A useful book describing this appalling reality is Bruce Arnold (2009), *The Irish Gulag – How the State Betrayed its Innocent Children*, Dublin: Gill & Macmillan.

The reality of the poor

In the global setting, the situation could not be more stark.[3] Almost half the world's population — over 3 billion people — live on less than $2.50 a day. At least 80 per cent of humanity lives on less than $10 a day. According to *The Millennium Development Goals Report 2011* one in five people and families on the planet (1.4 billion people) live on $1.25 a day. More than 80 per cent of the world's population live in countries where income differentials are widening. The poorest 40 per cent of the world's population accounts for only 5 per cent of global income. The richest 20 per cent accounts for three-quarters of world income. According to UNICEF, 22,000 children die *each day* due to poverty. They 'die quietly in some of the poorest villages on earth, far removed from the scrutiny and the conscience of the world. Being meek and weak in life makes these dying multitudes even more invisible in death'. Over a quarter of all children in developing countries are estimated to be underweight or stunted in development. Nearly a billion people entered the twenty-first century unable to read a book or sign their names. Various water problems affect at least half of humanity. Some 1.1 billion people in developing countries have inadequate access to water and 2.6 billion people lack basic sanitation.

Economic deprivation overlaps with, and accentuates, social exclusion and prejudice. This type of litany can go on and on. Let us just take the world's children. At least 1 billion of them live in material poverty. Of the 1.9 billion children from the developing world, 640 million are without adequate shelter, 400 million have no access to safe water and 270 million have no access to health services. In 2003, 10.6 million children died before they reached the age of five.[4] 1.5 million children die each year from lack of access to safe drinking water and adequate sanitation.

---

3   These data and illustrations are taken directly from *Poverty Facts and Stats* by Anup Shah, <http://www.globalissues.org/article/26/poverty-facts-and-stats>.

4   In Camus' novel *The Plague*, cited above, Dr Rieux says to Fr Paneloux following the death of the Othon child in the plague: '"And until my dying day I shall refuse to love a scheme of things in which children are put to torture."'

Approximately half the world's population now live in cities and towns. In 2005, one out of three urban dwellers (approximately 1 billion people) was living in slum conditions.

Is all of this the result of 'nature' or some inadequacy on the part of the poor? When we examine the distribution pattern of income and resources globally we can see that the world is characterized by extraordinary inequality, an inequality on an unthinkable, grotesque level. In 2005, the wealthiest 20 per cent of the world accounted for 76.6 per cent of total private consumption. The poorest 20 per cent accounted for just 1.5 per cent. The poorest 10 per cent accounted for 0.5 per cent and the wealthiest 10 per cent accounted for 59 per cent of all consumption. The total Gross Domestic Product of the forty-one most indebted poor countries (comprising 567 million people) is less than the wealth of the world's seven richest people. In the age of emperors and kings we knew who the powerful few were. Today, we have fewer 'emperors', with less visibility but with even more power. Fifty-one of the world's 100 wealthiest entities are private corporations.

Some might think that inequality, although still appalling, is reducing as 'modernity' and 'progress' advances. This is not so. An analysis of long-term trends shows that the wealth ratio differential between the richest and poorest countries was approximately:

- 3 to 1 in 1820
- 11 to 1 in 1913
- 35 to 1 in 1950
- 44 to 1 in 1973
- 72 to 1 in 1992

This gross inequality is not an accident. By the year 2000, the diversion of less than 1 per cent of the world's armaments expenditure to education spending would have permitted every child to have had access to schooling. Yet it did not happen. In fact, it would cost relatively little to address most of our real global problems. At the end of the twentieth century, in 1998, it would have cost $6 billion to provide education for all, $9 billion to provide water and sanitation for all and $13 billion to provide basic health and nutrition. It did not happen. But in the same year $8 billion was spent on cosmetics in the United States, $11 billion in ice cream in Europe, $12 billion on perfumes in Europe and the US and $17 billion on pet foods. Military spending in that year was $780 billion. The situation is no different today.

What kind of world is being described here? What kind of humanity is being revealed? It is not that people are necessarily evil or uncaring. They are not. On an interpersonal level most human beings are kind and considerate. The problem is that we are caught in a social structure that is *systemically* producing poverty and oppression. If we really want to care we therefore need to address our structural and systemic situation. From the perspective of the global poor – the vast majority of humanity – this situation must change. That is because it is producing dehumanization on an epic scale. Ours is a system that is producing not life but death.

What then of Ireland? In global terms we clearly belong to the wealthy minority. But poverty is relative. You are poor in relation to the society you live in. How does Irish society fare if we examine it from the perspective of the Irish poor? In Ireland the 'poor' are made up of overlapping categories. Perhaps 5,000 people are formally homeless. There are perhaps 30–40,000 Travellers, an ethnic minority who are despised or marginalized by most Irish people.[5] There are thousands of prisoners (15,425 were committed to prison in 2009), thousands of drug addicts, over 100,000 lone parents (38 per cent of whom are at risk of poverty), almost 6,000 inmates of direct provision accommodation for asylum seekers, and many thousands with physical and intellectual disabilities. Thousands of others suffer from chronic illness and mental distress. By the mid-2011, over 450,000 people were drawing unemployment welfare payments. At least 16 per cent of the population live in relative poverty (i.e. with incomes less than 60 per cent of the national median income). That's about 720,000 people. About 6.5 per cent of our population live in consistent poverty (i.e. lack consistently a number of basic material indicators for a comfortable average existence).

5   See Micheal McGréil, *Prejudice in Ireland Revisited* (1996) and *Pluralism and Diversity in Ireland* (2011).

That's about 290,000 people. Of the State's just over 1,000,000 children, 535,000 experienced poverty at some stage between 1994 and 2001, according to the ESRI.[6]

When we speak then of the poor and oppressed in Ireland, these are largely the people we are speaking about. These are the people who are most likely to seek integral social care. Micheál McGréil's recent study on prejudice in Ireland shows that drug addicts, alcoholics, Travellers and various non-Irish nationalities are among the most rejected and prejudiced against groups in our society.[7] For each individual there is a personal story but each also is the product of a wider socio-political framework that has either directly caused their social marginalization or has failed to resolve it. We need however to move beyond these quantitative lists to try and understand the implications for all of us of social inequality. Understanding these implications will show why it is that we need to respond with care and compassion to poverty and oppression rather than with indifference. The fact is that oppression does not just dehumanize the poor, it dehumanizes all of us.

The social implications of inequality

If we are genuinely committed to integral social care and compassion then we must become attentive not just to the reality but to the implications and meaning of this enormous social inequality. We can begin to think about this by considering a rather well-known quotation. It comes from Maev-Ann Wren's book *Unhealthy State – Anatomy of a Sick Society*:

---

6   For the most recent data on inequality and poverty in Ireland see the HEAP Report (2009) from Tasc and ICTU and Social Justice Ireland's 2011 Policy Briefing on Poverty.

7   M. McGréil (2011), *Pluralism and Diversity in Ireland*. See in particular Table 4.3.

Irish people die younger because they tolerate an inequality between them which breeds ill-health, and they accept a health care system and a view of health care which implicitly places lesser value on the lives of those with lesser means. (Wren: 2003: 50).

This is an extraordinary and disturbing sentence or, at least, it should be extraordinary and disturbing. After 2002/3, when her book was written, we had a further four years at least of unprecedented economic growth and prosperity. Does her judgement still ring true? Let us quote now from a more recent book – published in 2009 – by Sara Burke, which is provocatively entitled *Irish Apartheid – Healthcare Inequality in Ireland*.

We have an apartheid system of healthcare, where those who can afford to have quick access to what can be life-saving diagnosis and treatment, quicker than those who can't afford private care. This has always been the case but, in the last decade, the two-tier system of healthcare has been accentuated, with increasing numbers of people incentivised to take out private insurance, privileging them over those who cannot afford to skip the queue. (Burke 2009: 4)

Again, we can ask: what is going on here? What is being described in these books? Is this inequality and division simply the result of an administrative defect which results merely in inconvenience but little real harm? No, as we know, it is not. This structure of our health system has real implications. An extrapolation from a recent Institute of Public Health report *Inequalities in Mortality* (2001) has suggested that 5,400 people die prematurely each year in Ireland due to inequality and poverty. That amounts to more than 100 people each week, a figure so large it almost cannot be comprehended. It is only when this statistic becomes personalized around an individual – such as with Susie Long – that there is any political or media reaction. Susie Long died in October 2007. She chose to remain in the public health system rather than take out private health insurance. She died while on a lengthy waiting list for treatment. Has this reality changed? We know that it has not.

The pattern of illness and sickness in our society tells us something fundamental about our society. Equally, the social structure of our society – particularly the pattern of social inequality within it – tells us something fundamental about the causes and distribution of illness in our society. In other words, there is a clear and demonstrable connection between the pattern of illness and the pattern of social inequality. This connection is so close that we can say that social inequality is a health issue. It is far more than just that of course but it is absolutely a health issue as well. Extraordinarily, far from being a contentious claim, this is widely acknowledged and understood even by those who run our health service. For example, Dr John Kelleher, then Assistant National Director for Health Protection in the HSE, was quoted in *The Irish Times* in September 2006 as saying:

'The fundamental issue in relation to poor health is income; if you don't have that, you're never going to be healthy again.'

As we have shown above Ireland is a seriously unequal society. This, in turn, has a significant impact on the pattern of illness in our society. In simple terms, the greater the level of social inequality the greater the level of illness and the more unevenly distributed those illnesses are among the population. In short, the poor will be sicker and die younger in virtually all sickness categories than the wealthy.[8]

However, and this is important, social inequality is not a phenomenon that only has negative impacts on the poor and disadvantaged. Crucially, it has negative impacts for all in society. If we want a healthy and well functioning society, the most important and effective method by which this can be achieved is by creating and sustaining social equality.

It may be difficult for some people to think of Ireland as an unequal society. After all, we don't seem to have people starving on the streets. But poverty is always a relative concept. You are poor when measured relative to the norms within your given society. In aggregate terms we have been, and remain, a wealthy society. However, the critical factor in understanding poverty in a society is how that wealth is distributed. The key determinant in triggering social consequences and shaping the society is the distribution of that wealth – in other words, the real issue giving rise to social oppression is how big the gap is between the wealthy and the poor.

8   For data demonstrating this see K. Balanda and J. Wilde (2003), *Inequalities in Perceived Health – A Report on the All-Ireland Social Capital & Health Survey*, Institute of Public Health, Dublin.

Relative to the rest of the EU, particularly Western Europe, and relative to other aggregately wealthy societies, Ireland shows a very high level of social inequality. Only the United States consistently performs worse than Ireland in international terms among the top twenty wealthy societies. Bank of Ireland's *Wealth of the Nation Report* in 2007 showed that the wealthiest 1 per cent of the population owned 20 per cent of the country's wealth. The top 5 per cent owned 40 per cent of the nation's wealth. This means that the other 95 per cent of the population had the remaining 60 per cent of the country's wealth.

One internationally recognised measure of social equality is the Gini coefficient. This is a way of measuring income distribution. If all income went to 1 person and none to everyone else the coefficient would be 100. If everyone had the exact same income the coefficient would be 0. So, the lower the value, the more equal the society. In the mid-1980s Ireland's Gini coefficient was 33.1. In the mid-1990s it was 32.4. By 2000 it had improved to 30. However, by 2006 it had risen again to 32. This can be compared at the time to 23 in Sweden, 24 in Denmark and 28 in France, Germany and Norway.

The point is that over that twenty-year period – from the grim 1980s to the booming mid-noughties – our level of relative poverty and therefore social inequality remained largely unchanged. The data consistently shows that we are not a socially equal society. For example, the recently published *Hierarchy of Earnings, Attributes and Privileges Report* (HEAP, 2009), showed that in 2006 5 per cent of Irish households had a family income of €134,000 or more, while 26 per cent of households had an income of €20,000 or less. Overall, 58 per cent of households had a family income of €40,000 or less. This means that, at the height of the boom, when it was trumpeted that we were all wealthy, the fact was that almost 60 per cent of families had in fact relatively moderate incomes and at least a quarter were in real poverty. The top one-fifth of Irish income earners had incomes on average five times higher than the bottom one-fifth.

While these statistical ratios seem to indicate that inequality and poverty has remained relatively unchanged in Ireland over a twenty-year period, the reality is that the gap between the wealthy and the poor has widened significantly. If the aggregate level of income has risen in the society overall then, while the income differential ratio of 5:1 may remain the same, the gap has in fact become wider. A difference between €100 and €500 is €400 (5:1) but a difference between €200 and €1,000 is €800 (but still 5:1). This is what happened in Ireland during the Celtic Tiger period. Overall incomes doubled, the poverty ratios remained the same but the actual gap widened considerably.

The question that should trouble us further is whether we really want to create a society of social equality and care or whether those of us who are relatively comfortable and secure are happy with the way things are. Poverty seems to be invisible. It is rarely highlighted as a pressing social issue. It is rarely the stuff of heated political debates. It's almost as if poverty is not our concern. We need to understand that this is not so – social inequality affects us all.

To support this contention, I want to refer to Richard Wilkinson and Kate Pickett's interesting and important book *The Spirit Level – Why more equal societies almost always do better*. The argument of this book is straightforward and not by any means original. The authors set out to show that the benefits (both socially and in terms of health) of aggregate economic growth in rich countries have reached their limit. Now, the quality of life is determined they argue by the equal distribution of wealth.

What is particularly important about this book, however, is the impressive amount of empirical data that they present from around the world to support this argument. They show – I think compellingly – that income equality creates better outcomes across a whole range of social indicators. Specifically, they examine:

- Community life and social relations (social capital and trust)
- Mental health and drug use
- Physical health and life expectancy
- Obesity
- Educational performance
- Teenage births
- Violence
- Imprisonment
- Social mobility (opportunities).

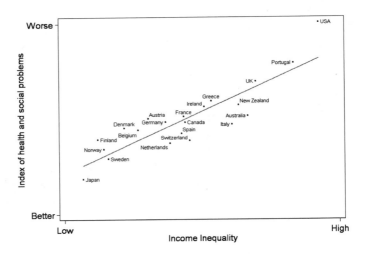

Figure Two: Correlation between Social Problems and Income Inequality.

(Source: Kate Wilkinson and Richard Pickett, *The Spirit Level*, 2009. See <http://www.equalitytrust.org.uk>)

They demonstrate that in rich countries health and social problems are closely related to the level of inequality in those countries. In short, the more unequal the society, the greater the extent of problems in these nine areas. It is a simple but elegant argument and one fully supported by the evidence. Figure Two summarises their data. The line trend demonstrates a clear correlation between various social problems and income inequality across a significant number of wealthy societies. In Ireland's case, the situation is slightly worse than the statistical model would have suggested.

Why might social equality be so important? The answer lies I think in understanding that we are fundamentally social beings who need to belong to the social groups within which we live. We have a compelling need to be accepted, to be able to participate, to be both able and free to access and utilize the resources of that society, whether they be material or symbolic. If we can't, if we are repulsed, marginalized, isolated, ill-treated or arbitrarily oppressed in any way, then it has devastating effects on us. To have *social distance* placed between you and the society to which you belong places you in an extremely unsettling position. These distances may be symbolic (the wrong accent, the wrong clothes) or actual (the wrong address, the wrong ethnicity) or, indeed, both. Where income differences are bigger, social distances (symbolic and actual) are greater. The materially and socially comfortable and the poor may live in the same country but they live in different social worlds.

For their part, Wilkinson and Pickett suggest that social inequality causes wider social problems because it leads to:

- A rise in anxiety
- Loss of self-esteem and social security
- Threats to the social self
- Loss of pride, increase in shame and loss of status
- Inequality increases social evaluation anxieties

Status and social acceptance are of critical importance for the type of social being that we humans are. Having low status has a direct and immediate impact on our well-being. It raises our stress levels, suppresses our immune levels and causes us anxiety. It makes us isolated, marginalized and reduced in our humanity. To quote Wilkinson and Pickett again: 'Chronic stress wears us down and wears us out.'[9]

Their argument is that social equality leads directly to social improvements in regards to each of their nine selected social indicators. It improves community life and social relations, improves mental and physical health, improves educational performance, reduces violence and the need for imprisonment and increases social opportunities and mobility. Hence, equal societies nearly always perform better.

The conclusion, I think, is clear. We need income and status equality in order to create socially and environmentally sustainable societies and, of course, to create healthy and caring societies. The point is that equality

9 See also in this connection contemporary research on social capital and social connections. See for example Robert Putnam (2000), *Bowling Alone: The Collapse and Revival of American Community*, New York: Simon & Schuster.

is a matter that should concern us all. We all live in society. The better that society is, the better for all of us. None of us can fruitfully exist as isolated and non-social beings unless we wish to live in a hyper-privatized world of private education, private hospitals, private security, private gated communities, etc. This surely is more a dystopian image of the world than something we might aspire to.

It seems apparent that when we are thinking about our society and about its health and well-being we are not thinking deeply enough. Our contemporary political debates are not at a deep enough level. In our present economic crisis, we are proceeding as if by reflex, driven by an accounting template of cutting services and raising taxes. In addition, crucial decisions, which will shape our society, are being made according to the power of various vested sectional interests to secure advantages for themselves but not necessarily according to the common good or the value of ensuring that we care for all. When this happens, the poor and weak lose – again.

What we don't have is a social plan which contains a vision for what type of country we want to have. We have apparently economic-based plans centred on a 'smart economy'. What about a social plan centred on a 'just and equal society'? Especially if it turns out that a smart society is in fact a just and equal society. The bottom line is that achieving social equality is not just about the poor – it's about all of us. We all benefit. The Foreword of the HEAP Report states:

> Ireland is now in the midst of both an economic crisis and a deepening equality crisis, and the danger is that only tackling the economic crisis will increase the inequality gap which already exists. The reality is we cannot afford not to address inequality. On the contrary, we need to assert equality as a core societal value – as a benchmark against which to test and refine any proposed responses to recession. There is certainly a need for changes in expenditure and taxation but there is no reason why such changes cannot be implemented in a way which reduces rather than reinforces inequality.
>
> There is both a moral and an economic case for advancing equality. Equality should be a core value because it underpins the human dignity and worth of all individuals.
>
> The desire for greater equality is reflected in a 2009 Behaviour and Attitudes poll commissioned by TASC, showing that 72 per cent of adults are concerned at

the level of wealth inequality in Ireland while 85 per cent believe the government should take steps to reduce income inequality.

Living in a more equal society has been found to benefit everyone, not just people previously living in poverty. Furthermore, research has shown that organisational mechanisms to promote equality and diversity enhance productivity, innovation and employee retention. Income inequality has been identified as a causal factor for low life expectancy, poor educational attainment, high levels of violence and lower levels of social mobility. All of this evidence illustrates that promoting equality must play a central role in developing an effective response to economic recession.

Therefore, quite apart from our claims regarding the humanizing effect on all of us of practising integral care and compassion, even enlightened self-interest should also lead us to create a socially equal society and world. Once again it can be seen that our conceptions of what is genuinely in our own interest are seriously narrow and flawed.

Having considered all of the above, can we now bring these ideas and implications together in a number of propositions which might guide the direction of compassionate activism in the socio-political dimension? The following outline five possible such propositions. As in Chapter Four, where we drew on the insights of Carl Rogers, so here we will rely on some of the ideas proposed by Paulo Freire.

Integral social care practice in the socio-political dimension

Proposition 1: Integral social care should view socio-political reality from the perspective of the poor and oppressed

There are a number of reasons why this might be so. First, one must view social reality from some standpoint. There is no truly 'objective', pure view which offers a detached, scientific perspective. In truth, each social actor is always engaged in the world and always reproduces it or contests it. There is no neutrality. As even the great natural scientist Charles Darwin said: 'How odd it is that anyone should not see that all observation must be for or against some view if it is to be of any service.' Choosing to see the social world from the perspective of the poor is merely to see it from the perspective of the global majority. It is to make our position clear and to make explicit our commitment to care and justice. As integral social carers we are in any event thrown up against the world of the poor and oppressed. Many social care workers come themselves of course from the world of the poor. But whether we are poor or marginalized ourselves or not, if we see those with whom we work as objects and not as subjects with their own perspective then we become potentially part of the structure of oppression. Far better to stand with them and try and see what they see. We cannot avoid making the choice as to where we stand.

Secondly, as we have argued in this chapter, the very existence of the poor and oppressed provide an empirical measure of the claims of modernity to deliver progress, human rights, justice, equality, liberty and democracy for all. The scandal of their existence calls these claims into question and demands that an account be made. They expose the truth of our socio-political world and blow away the illusions and mythologies which delude and entrance us. Seeing from their perspective provides a better epistemological and phenomenological foundation to see the social world as it truly is.

Finally, their existence challenges our common humanity. Do we really care? Do we really have compassion? They call us to respond and, by responding, to recover our common humanity. A world in which the majority suffers from basic wants, in which our fellow human beings suffer needlessly, is inhuman. It diminishes us all. Do we want our conception of our humanity to be implicitly defined by its systemic indifference to the oppressions of others?

Proposition 2: If we see from the perspective of the poor, we see injustice, poverty and oppression

The reality of the poor and oppressed reveals a socio-political world of continuing and worsening injustice. It reveals a social reality that does not change – the poor remain and do not 'progress'. Those who are 'below', on the 'underside of history', remain socially marginalized and diminished. While liberation has occurred in some categories it has been reduced in others. The present economic crisis in capitalism has left more in the poor Southern world deprived of essential resources and more in the developed world itself deprived of basic social services. If you have no social resource needs, and sufficient private means to meet all your requirements, then the world continues to present itself as functional and successful. But if you have needs and are dependent on the wider society to help you because you lack the material or symbolic resources to meet your requirements, then the world appears harsh and unforgiving. From the perspective of the poor, ours can be a sick and cruel social world.

Proposition 3: Because of this, the socio-political world must change

Once we take account of the empirical reality of poverty and oppression (and indeed of the ecological crisis before us also) it is clear that this socio-political reality must change. It must change because we are failing to realize our common humanity. Rather than humanizing ourselves we are dehumanizing not only the oppressed but ourselves as well. We live in the midst of a catastrophic failure of compassion. We are all failing to bring about the better world which is within our power to do. We are trapped by a system which is forcing us to be indifferent to each other. As has been shown, it is in all our interest to achieve a society and world of equality and maximum freedom. We need to recover our humanity through the exercise of integral care and compassion. We need to do this because poverty and oppression kills. The poor are dying before their time.

Proposition 4: In order to realize our common humanity, we need a society of basic needs for all rather than of wealth for a few

We cannot of course ensure that every person is absolutely equal in all respects. That is not what is being proposed here. It would be both impossible and unnecessary. What is at issue is bringing about a social world in which all basic human needs are met, particularly food, shelter, healthcare and education. That is perfectly realizable. But to bring it about may require some of us, the global minority, to share and cede some of our material advantages. We cannot all live the lifestyle of the wealthy Western consumer. It simply cannot be done if for no other reason than that there are not the resources available on the planet to permit it. By therefore consuming according to this lifestyle, we are explicitly oppressing our fellow human beings who as a direct consequence are left with fewer resources. By taking more than our fair share we are leaving less for others. It is however possible to bring about the universal satisfaction of basic needs once there is the requisite socio-political commitment to human care and solidarity. The attainment of this vision is the ultimate goal of integral social care and the purposeful practice of compassionate activism. A society based on manic and dysfunctional wealth accumulation by the few offers us no basis for bringing about a humanized and humanizing civilization for all.

Proposition 5: The poor carry key values which can help to bring this about

The poor and oppressed should not be mere objects of our work and care. They are subjects in their own right with their own view of the world. They too are integral social carers. They are the key agents of social transformation because their very existence demands that social reality change. Their own capacity to survive and endure, despite their oppression, demonstrates that they carry critical values of resilience and solidarity which are essential for any humanizing project. It is a remarkable observation that almost everyone who works with, and shares time with, those who are poor, whether they be the economically poor, or a cultural minority, or people with a physical or intellectual disability or distress, whether they be at home or abroad, come to acknowledge that they have received far more than they have given and have found themselves transformed by their relationships. The great joy of integral social care relationships lies in this mutual transformation, this mutual humanization. The poor are not therefore passive receivers – they too are active agents of change. For this reason, we who may not come directly from this reality ourselves, need to be attentive to them and learn from them. Contrary to our conventional scale of utility, which regards value as a product of wealth and status, the poor and oppressed transmit humanizing values of the utmost importance. They call us to our better visions of ourselves, both personally and socially. They are the bearers of utopian hope, the hope that we can create a society that includes all and provides basic needs for all. Thus, they are the creators and foundation of a civilization of integral care and compassion.

Our proposal is that these five propositions can serve to orientate integral social care practice in the socio-political dimension. However, we must take note and acknowledge that, despite straightforwardly presenting these propositions, nothing here is 'proved'. Nothing is conclusive. Much, perhaps all, of what is asserted here is contestable. That, of course, is in the nature of political claims. We should not be troubled or angry at that. We should make no claim to moral superiority or demand conformity with our 'programmes' for change. At the end of the day, one is free to choose the world one wants. Instead, we should dedicate ourselves to constant dialogue and engagement in order to argue for a transformed world based on reason and compassion. A new society and world characterized by integral care can never be forced. That would be a contradiction in terms and would defeat its very purpose. Therefore, while our ultimate focus should be on bringing about a society and world where every human being is cared for in all their dimensions, our immediate practice must be necessarily grounded on compassionate and liberating relationships. We should be committed to an incremental but determined *process* of integral political change brought about by the means of dialogue and conscientization. The *outcome* will then take care of itself.

In the final part of this book, I wish to outline in brief terms what such a compassionate activism might look like in practice. The challenge to be faced now is how to translate the claims and assertions presented thus far into an achievable and workable *living practice*. We will suggest that a dialogic practice offers one possible sensible and humanizing methodology to bring about genuine and radical personal and social transformation. This is an approach available to all whether they are a professional social carer or not. In summary, the proposal will be that dialogic practice offers an ethic and mode of living for everyone.

PART FOUR

Integral Liberation

Towards Dialogic Practice

Based on the overwhelming reality of inequality, poverty and deprivation, and of our mounting ecological crisis, it seems clear that our present
socio-political system is not working. It is producing antagonisms within
societies, between countries and between humanity and our planet. We
are all caught up in the effects of these antagonisms. Some of us may think
we are immune but we are not. Sooner or later, the consequences of these
dysfunctions will strike all of us. If we are poor and living in the wrong part
of the social world, they have struck us already.

The problem that we have is systemic in character. It is not the result
of some elementary flaw in human nature. Most human beings are fundamentally decent and good and respond to human need and suffering at a
personal level in ways that are caring and compassionate. As Bill Mollison
has pointed out, there has always been an 'ethical majority'.[1] We must
remind ourselves of this even in the face of so much horror and destruction so that we do not lose hope or mistakenly imagine ourselves as worse
than we really are. The fact is that we are caught in the confines of a social
structure oriented towards wealth accumulation and consumerism. We are
doing harm without thought, without consideration and often without
any awareness of what we are doing.

Our political and economic systems are configured to ensure continual
economic growth and maximum exploitation of resources. Economistic
ideas and standards of competitiveness, efficiency and instrumental rationality have become the unquestionable criteria for measuring good human

---

1   See Bill Mollison (1997), *Introduction to Permaculture*, Tasmania: Tagari
    Publications.

social behaviour and are socially constructed to be the values and practices which will lead to optimum human well-being.

This system is broken. The most recent economic crisis has shown that it is not working even according to its own logic. Unregulated free marketization has lead to a financial crash of historic proportions and has caused banking and financial service crises throughout the world. However, as always, it is the poor who pay disproportionably for this either through further taxes or wage cuts or through the contraction of public services. The erosion of public finances and the huge deficits run by most states has led to the further withdrawal of the State from much-needed social service provision. Those in need of care must either wait or do without.

What we need are solutions. We need a system that produces harmonies not antagonisms. This is our historical challenge – to re-design our socio-political system so that it produces harmonies between human beings and between humanity and our planet. Achieving harmony – social and ecological – is the political cause of today. It is within this wider socio-political context that we must ground our understanding of contemporary integral social care and locate the practices of compassionate activism.

I think this project of re-design in favour of social and ecological harmony can begin now. Indeed, it is already underway in places and communities all around the world.[2] Central to it is building new culture from the bottom-up based on dialogue and participation. New ideas, new businesses and new modes of exchange between people are emerging and re-emerging from the old, decaying model. It is in this sense that we might now be at a time of hope. However, to really enhance this momentum we need to make it explicit and visible and make clear that a new model is being born. It is as yet incremental, tentative and without a blueprint. What it has is an objective and a method. We need to openly commit to it and place its realization at the centre of our compassionate activism. We need a system that places integral social care at its heart and not as an add-on extra.

2   See for example the website of Feasta, The Foundation for the Economics of Sustainability, for details and links to this vibrant emergence of ideas and projects: <http://www.feasta.org>.

In this chapter I will try and describe some of the key elements in how we might bring about systemic change in our integral social care methodologies and, by extension, in the wider social world. In the previous chapter we provided a critique of the present social and political system. There should be no critique without a positive proposal. Below is outlined one such proposal, not presented as an exclusive imperative but offered as one possible method which places dialogue at its centre. The political and professional methodology for integral carers must be a *dialogic practice* because such a practice is most consistent and reflective of integral care's core values of acceptance, mutuality and humanization. It is also consistent with the most important political idea of all – democracy. Dialogic practice also permits us to unite means and ends and process and outcome. Dialogic practice lies squarely within the thinking and legacy of both Carl Rogers and Paulo Freire and permits us to combine insights and knowledge from both.

However, before describing this viable and practical approach, we need to briefly examine once again the outlines of the social care model that we need to replace.

The model that we need to replace

As we have noted earlier in this book one of the central discourses of our present model is 'person-centredness'. In most institutional settings social care practitioners, managers and administrators pay formal acquiescence to person-centredness as a set of values and as a professional practice. This discourse suggests that the needs of the individual service user should determine the specific services they receive and that the individual should exercise control over those services. In addition, it asks what is possible for the individual to achieve in the social world immediately about them rather than asking what is available for them to achieve based on the range of 'care services' actually accessible to them. In short, according to this discourse, individual need, as determined by the individual him or herself, should determine the service provided rather than it being the available service menu which decides what is possible.[3]

However, the fact of the matter is that genuine person-centredness rarely occurs in practice. In a study into the quality and effectiveness of services to people with a physical disability in County Mayo conducted in 2007, I found that 'in none of the effectiveness indicators outlined in the questionnaire does a majority of total respondents report that the service they receive meets their needs "very or quite" well'.[4] The Executive Summary reported that:

> The real need identified by many focus group and interview participants is for relationships, the continuity of their social networks and enhanced social inclusion. Service coverage is reported as not an end in itself but as a means to secure personal empowerment, fulfillment and autonomy. The study finds that perhaps the greatest quality and effectiveness deficit lies in the provision of relationships and social inclusion to people with disabilities. This finding suggests that service users are seeking the provision, or the further enhancement, of a social, or person-centred model of service, rather than an overtly medical model.

Genuinely achieving person-centredness in social care provision is curtailed by a range of factors. A number of justifications are offered which seek to explain the difficulty of achieving it. The first and most obvious is resource limitation. Not everything can be done for the individual because not everything that is required can be afforded. Hence, a service menu must be put in place and selections confined to that.

Secondly, service organizations, whether they are State or voluntary, are not organizationally configured to deliver a person-centred service. Instead, they are designed around 'programmes', plans and the organizational and

---

3   For excellent descriptions of person-centred planning see the outstanding work of John O'Brien and Herbert Lovett, for example *Finding a Way Toward Everyday Lives: The Contribution of Person Centered Planning* (1999), Harrisburg, PA: Pennsylvania Office of Mental Retardation.

4   This study was conducted through a self-answering questionnaire distributed to the approximately 1,000 people on the disability register in County Mayo. A number of focus groups were also held. The report, conducted independently of, but commissioned by, the HSE, was presented to them in 2008.

professional roles and competencies of their staff. Developing and improving their service menu appears to be the tangible sign of effectiveness and development. Funding applications and provision are often determined by the type of programmes that are available either for tendering or for delivery. In addition, funding criteria are usually determined by specific modes of service provision and planning and the receipt of funding is often tied to predetermined performance targets and output measurables. The result is that organizations are largely institutionally and culturally incapable of reducing their power and surveillance over services in favour of genuine person-centred service provision. Funding and performance measurable criteria, endemic to the contemporary ideology of managerialism and performance management, dictate a command and control culture and structure rather than a support and enabling function. The result is an inevitable focus on *service coverage* rather than on *integral relationship*. The attention of organizations becomes focused on enhancing service delivery efficiency rather than on ensuring that services are specifically tailored to each user *as determined by* that user.

Finally, the onslaught of these various forms of 'new managerialism' has served to deeply augment and reinforce the focus on coverage and outputs rather than on relationship and facilitation. As Bronwyn Davies has defined (citing Rose 1999) new managerialism 'is characterised by the removal of the locus of power from the knowledge of practising professionals to auditors, policy-makers and statisticians, none of whom need know anything about the profession in question' (Davies 2003: 91). As we have discussed earlier in this book, it is predicated upon a *de facto* distrust of the working professional who is regarded as, without rigorous management and performance surveillance, unlikely to meet pre-determined targets and outputs. That the professional may in fact question the efficacy or value of these targets and outputs merely further establishes their untrustworthiness in principle. The professional practitioner is regarded as not having access to the privileged knowledge that must guide the manager. The assumption and assertion made is that the manager knows and the worker must do as they are instructed. The service user is even further removed from consideration. It is the manager who occupies the role of greatest importance because it is they who are confronting and in contact with true 'reality'.

It is they who must engage with the economically dictated constraints of what is possible. Within this logic, professionals and service users may well all agree about what is desirable but it is the manager who is the link and conduit with the 'real world' where only some things, sometimes, are possible. The rationale for the manager's role and responsibilities is thus 'reality' itself, and with 'reality' no argument is possible.

> Within the terms of the new system individuals will be presented with an (often overwhelming) range of pressing choices and administrative tasks for which they are responsible. But any questioning of the system itself is silenced or trivialised. The system itself is characterised as both natural and inevitable. Resistance to it by individuals (and that includes critiques such as this) is constituted as ignorance of what the 'real' (financial) 'bottom-line' issues are, as sheer cussedness, or as a sign reminding management of individual workers' replaceability. (Davies 2003: 93)

Leaving aside for now the observation that all social reality is constructed and subject to change – in other words all 'reality' is created to be so – one of the implications of this model is that the achieving of the predetermined targets becomes ends in themselves. Whether these targets are of any real value is rarely to be considered. Once the objectives are in place and the strategies for their management and surveillance established, the nature and inherent value of the work quickly becomes of lesser relevance. If the targets are met then the work must have been successful. Once it is up and running, the individual service user's capacity to re-configure this structure is minimal. Indeed, more likely than not, they are largely rendered invisible and silenced under the weight of this rationalized logic.[5]

As George Ritzer has shown, for these bureaucratized, rationalized systems to work and deliver efficiency, calculability, predictability and control, the human element has to be constrained. After all, it is people with their peculiar needs and sensibilities that are the greatest threat to the smooth running of any system.

---

5   Interestingly, the growth of new managerialism is now so pervasive it has also reshaped contemporary Third Level education which has become increasingly characterized by disconnected, 'bite-sized' modules and 'intended learning outcomes'.

These three overlapping and reinforcing factors indelibly shape our system of social care provision. In addition, adding to each of these factors, we are also experiencing a growing privatization of social care provision. In Ireland this is particularly evident in childcare, fostering services and in care of the elderly. A 'for profit' social care service cannot but conceptualize care as a commodity and is inevitably subject to financial performance criteria which can only further accentuate the managerial processes outlined above.

However, that is not to say that worthwhile and authentic work does not get done within our existing system. Of course it does. I do not wish to exaggerate or caricature the present model and deliberately create a 'straw man'. There is much in present practice which is excellent and to be valued and many individual managers are of course outstanding in their roles and effort despite enormous challenges. However, much of this achievement occurs *in spite* of the prevailing system not *because* of it and is the result of the ongoing dedication and commitment of so many professional social care practitioners. Most of these I believe would recognize the features of the system that we have just outlined.

There is nothing new under the sun so therefore proposing that there can be an entirely new system is to propose too much. Instead, we need to build on all of the positive features of current practice. In particular, we need to genuinely operationalize person-centredness as a philosophy and methodology and we need to re-frame our working procedures away from command and control and onto support and enabling. To do this effectively we need to radically reconfigure our integral care approach.

Towards a new model of dialogic practice

The imperative to create a new model of integral care that impacts positively not just on specifically categorized cohorts of service users but on the wider society generally is that the present model is not working. As has been argued above, the socio-political system is dysfunctional because it is causing antagonisms which harm us all. The social care system is not working because it is not delivering a genuine person-centred, liberating model. In both settings, we are failing to fully dedicate ourselves to bringing about maximum humanization.

It is clear that what we need are solutions. Yet solutions seem to be in short supply and, insofar as any are being offered, they all appear to be in the realm of macro, 'big-picture' structural changes which only governments can bring about. Hence, we wait frustrated and disempowered while our 'leaders' in reality strive to maintain the *status quo*. Yet the interesting thing is that the solution to many of our problems can best be found through a radical 'bottom-up', participative, dialogic process. Not only is this the most comprehensive way to deal with our problems and fix them, but it would also re-invigorate our democratic and social culture. What we want to do after all is to build harmonies and find solutions, and not accentuate antagonisms and build conflict and despair. This dialogic practice approach also offers a new and reinvigorated role for the integral social carer as a pedagogical facilitator rather than as a 'fixer' of social problems.

Thus, the method of dialogic practice is proposed in response to two sets of overlapping challenges. The first is how do we deliver social care (understood in as wide a manner as possible) in a way that is most humanizing and effective? The second is how do we bring about progressive social change in a similarly humanizing and effective way?

Seizing upon dialogue as central to this is not to make a unique or original claim. On the contrary, the importance of dialogue is grounded in the perspective we have presented throughout which we have drawn from a diverse range of thinkers. Thus, Rogers asserts that 'Good communication, free communication, with or between men, is always therapeutic' (1989: 333). We have already cited Freire's dictum that 'Dialogue is thus an existential necessity' (1986: 61) and Bakhtin's that '... authentic human life is the open-ended dialogue. Life by its very nature is dialogic' (1984: 293). The great Jewish philosopher Martin Buber reminds us that 'A person makes his appearance by entering into relation with other persons' (1984: 62).

Meaningful, open and genuine dialogue is the route to, and the manifestation of, our humanity. Being listened to and being responded to constitute the beginning of forging a liberating and humanizing relationship and, by extension, a more compassionate culture. Central to dialogic practice is the acknowledgement of the voice and identity of the other person and of their unique and valuable perspective on themselves and the world. The purpose of dialogic practice is to give people themselves the power and right to both *define and solve* their own problems.

There are a number of key principles that underline this approach. First, it recognizes that *process* (how we do what we do) is as important as the *outcome*. This principle is consistent with all that has been argued above. Secondly, it explicitly asserts that people can be *trusted* to make the right decision. In this sense, it affirms genuine democracy and declares that people do not have to be manipulated or 'managed' into responsible behaviour. Thirdly, it is democratic. It recognizes the identity and voices of all and does not privilege the 'expert' or 'professional' over others. Finally, it acknowledges that dialogue is a mode of discovery of both the self and the world. We discover who we are by the process of dialogue – of word and response – with others and we come to know reality itself through naming and understanding our shared social experience.

Contra the cult of managerialism, what we require is the prioritizing and valuing of humanization as determined by each person and service user and not necessarily as determined by pre-set performance targets. Humanization is the outcome of our integral care practice and is achieved through a process that itself humanizes, i.e. a process of open mutual dialogue based on non-judgemental acceptance that permits the person to exercise the greatest possible human freedom and choice. What we need to do as integral carers is to work with people to solve life's problems. We want to build harmonies and solutions, not antagonisms and grievances. We want to maximize human liberation for all. In our dialogic practice we come to discover the uniqueness and value of the other person, their worldview and circumstances, and their assessment of what they require for a full human existence. The role of the carer – be they a designated professional or otherwise – is to facilitate that liberation. This may also involve them entering into further dialogic interaction with the wider socio-political world in order to achieve integral transformation. In this sense, because it both captures an effective process and a set of values, dialogic practice is the appropriate method of compassionate activism.

Outlining a dialogic process for integral care

This approach of dialogic practice can be described in terms of its goals, its assumptions and its methodology.

First, the goal of integral social care should be clearly formulated. This is an essential prerequisite for effective practice. After all, in order to get somewhere we need to know where we are trying to go. The specific goal/s should be determined by the service user themselves in dialogue with the integral carer. A renewed social care practice must also be based on a clear statement of fundamental purpose. Such a clear purpose would in turn permit both integral carers and service users to have a yardstick to truly appraise the efficacy of their relationship. A clear statement of value should also provide the integral carer with the conviction and standard to challenge bad practice and social injustice.

Throughout this book we have argued that the ultimate purpose of integral social care is the humanization of the person and that this humanization begins in a non-judgemental, authentic relationship. The process of humanization extends from the interpersonal domain into the socio-political. Humanization must also embrace the carer.

Understanding our ultimate goal as humanization permits us to orientate ourselves around what is really important and what we really need to achieve in our social care practice. We need to assist each person, including ourselves, to discover their own true self and to be free to be themselves through the exercise of free choices and decisions. Anything that dehumanizes people must be resisted. Consequently, the integral carer must ensure that they are on the side of humanity in their values and their practices.

Thus, in working specifically with an individual or a group the first and primary question to be posed in a new solutions-focused dialogic methodology is: what is it that you need in order to be more human? This is the opening and generating question that should frame all our authentic relationships. The other person is the only one who can answer that on their own behalf. It is *their* answer that determines the orientation of the relationships and determines the objectives and 'targets' to be met. After all, it is their humanization that is in issue. Only by posing and by being attentive to this question can we be truly responsive to the specificities and circumstances of each person. This is far more appropriate and safer than to assume that our service menus meet the needs of certain predetermined care categories such as 'disabled' people, Travellers, drug users and so on. Each person is a unique and valuable individual and not the exemplar of a category. They should not be reduced to types in such a way as to say 'every wheelchair user is ... or needs ...' The happiness and well-being of each person is something to be always uniquely identified and discovered in a mutual human relationship with that particular person.

In summary then the task of a new, reinvigorated system of care is to construct a methodology that is more responsive to people and their real, self-identified needs. The way to do this is to give people the power to define and solve their own problems. In this manner, the means and ends become harmonized, i.e. the means used lead to the ends desired.

Second, the core assumption underlying this new model of care is that those affected by issues are the best sources of knowledge about what needs to be done. This includes both the individual at the heart of the issue and their immediate family and/or social network. They may not be the *only* sources but they are the *best* sources. We must enable them to go and address those issues. They are the experts in their own affairs. What they need from integral social carers is not an assertion of the carer's superior expertise, or privileged knowledge, but support and facilitation. This assumption, if truly internalized as a value, repositions the balance of power between the integral carer and the service user. It is the service user and their direct social network who are the experts and the carer who is the learner and supporter. Thus the integral carer's role is to provide maximum knowledge, information and control to the service user so that it is they who are best equipped to make decisions and formulate targets. This description of the role of the integral social carer acts as a necessary corrective to the possibility that professionalization might lead to distance and superiority.

Therefore, we need to acknowledge that people can be trusted and empowered. Those affected by issues, or those at the frontline of issues, are the best judges of what needs to be done. We should permit them to act.

This involves ceding power and control from centralized, bureaucratized systems. We need to allow all kinds of individuals and groups – be they community groups, various citizen groups, disability groups, drug addicts, even practitioners in the frontline of new businesses and public services – to work out their own solutions from the bottom up.

Third, this assumption in turn suggests a straightforward working methodology. There is nothing novel or original about this methodology. It is grounded in Rogers' concept of non-judgemental acceptance and Freire's proposals regarding dialogue and conscientization. It is the working method of any progressive community development programme. However, this method of dialogic practice needs to be extended radically to bring about a genuine bottom-up approach to providing and experiencing integral social care. Social care should be understood as holistically as possible. The methodology of dialogic practice derives from the working assumption that the affected group or individual defines the problem and decides what they need to do to address it.[6]

There are five identifiable steps in this method. At each step, the integral social carer should be a facilitator and supporter. The first step is for the affected or relevant individual or group to develop a generating question around the defined problematic. By a generating question I mean a question designed to generate answers. In other words, we need to translate problems into questions. Thus, for example, a group might ask how can we as people with physical disabilities better succeed in living independently. How can we as a community better reduce the number of drug users in our area? How can I as an individual, despite my various personal and structural constraints, better become who I want to be? Framing the question oneself, out of one's own life world and experience, allows one to be a subject who is capable of acting on one's own personal and social reality.

---

6   It needs to be noted here that 'social care' encompasses a very wide variety of activities and domains of practice and that it is essential that specific dialogic methods be developed to ensure effectiveness in each of these domains. Thus how one dialogues with children, with refugees, with ethnic groups all vary greatly. What is being proposed in this chapter is a general methodological outline.

The second step is to permit the affected individual or group to generate their own answers. The integral carer becomes an enabler, a facilitator of this process, but not the 'expert'. Answers are generated through authentic, open dialogue between the individual concerned, their families, supporters and social networks, or among the participants in the wider affected group with the integral carer as simply one further contributor. There are many sophisticated methods in existence for creating dialogue and exchange. We do not need to elaborate them here but they include using structured meetings, open source interactions, 'world café' gatherings, use of various internet-based facilities, open and anticipation dialogues and so on. It may take time for the 'culture of silence' to be overcome but storytelling, drama, art, music and various Freirean 'coding' methods can all be hugely helpful. The point is to give time in order to allow people to find their voice, to speak their own words and to uncover who they are in the process. It may be slow and it may be 'inefficient' but a commitment to authentic dialogue is an inherent part of the humanization process. Methods can readily be developed to ensure that everyone participates in such dialogic processes and not just the dominant and articulate. Equally, systems can be designed to permit those who cannot speak (those with intellectual disabilities and otherwise) and those who are rarely permitted to speak (such as children and non-citizens) to participate in a meaningful manner. The problem does not lie in whether there are the means to do it. The problem lies only in whether there is the will.

Third, in developing answers individuals and groups need to be given the mechanisms of control to implement those answers. Thus resource allocation planning and budgetary allocations need to be devolved directly to those affected by these decisions. Participatory planning and budget construction can readily be done by groups themselves. They can decide priorities and schedules. They should be trusted to do so.

Fourth, the individuals and groups should be accountable for their actions. It is in fact dehumanizing to hold so-called 'disadvantaged' groups to a lesser standard of performance than should otherwise be the case with similar peer groups. This has frequently happened with certain categories of people such as those with physical disabilities. If you make a decision you should be responsible.

Finally, therefore, affected individuals and groups can design systems for reviewing and rechecking experiences, decisions and priorities. This means continual reflection on practice and performance as it directly impacts on the affected subjects themselves. Thus, they should exercise maximum control but should also be accountable and self-critical. In human affairs there is always conflict and always error and this needs to be addressed and handled not denied. Because we always get something wrong and can never be perfect we need to continually reflect and relearn.

The consequence of this approach is that professionals and organizations need to redefine their roles and place themselves at the service of this liberatory process. This means that their key task becomes one of distributing knowledge, exchanging information and skills and facilitating the humanization process. This should significantly reduce the tendency to bureaucratization and top-down management systems. This in turn should permit the development of truly smart and responsive organizations, orientated around *service response* rather than *service coverage*. These new organization structures should in turn better manifest, encourage and support the dialogic practice of integral social care.

In summary then, what is proposed here is that we should orientate our practice around responding to our real, human needs for relationships and freedom; that those affected by issues are the best sources of knowledge about what needs to be done; and that a simple methodology of practice facilitates, through authentic dialogue, those affected by an issue themselves developing generating questions, discovering their own answers and implementing those answers through an accountable devolution of power and resources. Dialogic practice requires time, non-judgemental acceptance, real communication centred on listening and authentic response and the willingness to meet each other on the plain of our common humanity through the recognition of our shared vulnerabilities and needs. In this way, the people at the heart of our care can engage in a humanizing process that allows them to be subjects in the world and better permits them to attain the outcome of humanization itself.

In conclusion, then, an outline of the methodology is as follows:

Purpose
- Giving people the power to define and solve their own problems

Principles
- The process is as important as the outcome
- People can be trusted to make the right decision
- Democracy should characterize our practice
- Dialogue is a mode of discovery of self and the world

Goals
- Goals must be clear
- Humanization as an ultimate goal
- Goals are to be set by subjects themselves in dialogue and are outlined in a Specific Generating Question which emerges in the dialogue – *What is it that we need in order to ... ?*

Core assumption
- Those affected by issues are the best sources of knowledge about what needs to be done

Working methodology
- Develop in dialogue a generating question around a defined problematic
- Facilitate the person or group to generate answers
- Provide/source the tools and resources to permit the person or group to implement their answers
- The person or group is accountable
- Learn, reflect and re-do

Dialogic practice needs
- Time
- Non-judgmental acceptance
- Real communication – genuine listening and authentic response
- The meeting place of our common humanity

Implications for professional practice

- Social care practitioners become facilitators of the humanization process
- An orientation around service response rather than service coverage
- Central skill becomes relationship-formation and the capacity and willingness to enter into dialogue

If communities and organizations – both real and virtual, across all social fields – could configure themselves in this way we would see a real social, political and cultural renewal. Our people would stop being made dependent and would start acting. We would build a culture of engagement, one that hopefully would sweep away our discredited political system based on clientalism and dependency. Our organizations would become facilitators of liberation not depositories of limited resources unequally distributed.

What is outlined here is not utopian. It is eminently achievable. One particularly fascinating example of the use of open dialogue has been the work of Jaakko Seikkula and his colleagues in the mental health services in Lapland in Northern Finland. In his fascinating book, co-written with Tom Erik Arnkill, *Dialogical Meetings in Social Networks*,[7] he describes how he discovered almost by accident the therapeutic efficacy of open dialogue in responding to people with first-episode psychotic outbreaks. He and his team quickly realized the crucial value of dialogue itself in assisting people to make sense of their problems and bringing about full recovery. In the open dialogue method the individual with mental distress meets with their family, their key supporters and a number of professional therapists to freely discuss their problems without an agenda or pre-determined outcome.[8]

---

7   J. Seikkula and T. E. Arnkil (2006), *Dialogical Meetings in Social Networks*, London and New York: Karnac.

8   See the inspiring documentary made on this called *Open Dialogue – An Alternative Finnish Approach to Healing Psychoses* (2011) by the American therapist and documentary maker Daniel Mackler. For more information on this go to <http://www.iraresoul.com>.

This dialogic approach, which rests on a number of key principles, has had demonstrably better results than approaches based on medication or more traditional forms of therapy. These principles include the tolerance of uncertainty ('As part of this approach, the question that a crisis poses, What shall we do? is kept open until the collective dialogue itself produces a response or dissolves the need for action' (Seikkula 2003: 408)); dialogism; and polyphony ('the dialogical emphasis is on generating multiple expressions, with no attempt to uncover a particular truth' (*ibid*: 410)).

Seikkula's direct experiences of the merits of open dialogue have granted him rich insights into its wider efficacy.

> For as I see it, dialogue is not a method; it is a way of life. We learn it as one of the first things in our lives, which explains why dialogue can be such a powerful happening. Because it is the basic ruling factor of life, it is in fact very simple. It is its very simplicity that seems to be the paradoxical difficulty. It is so simple that we cannot believe that the healing element of any practice is simply to be heard, to have response, and that when the response is given and received, our therapeutic work is fulfilled. Our clients have regained agency in their lives by having the capability for dialogue. (Seikkula 2011: 185)

Of course there are many organizations who must necessarily engage with people who are chronically incapacitated and require direct care and protection. But in all instances people need to be treated as subjects with their own unique voice. The type of orientation suggested here is entirely achievable once people have the confidence and the impetus to change the way we are doing things. Fundamental to this is to restore our belief in people and to trust them with the power to do the right thing.

Dialogic practice provides an approach to achieve personal, economic, social and political change that is radical but uses no jargon, involves no protest, is positive, smart and empowering and uses tools already available. It centres on bottom-up participative solution seeking and radical democratization both as an available methodology and a set of working values. It offers a model for addressing other issues besides those traditionally identified with social care. Indeed, it offers us a way out of our present phase of 'post-democracy' by which we have the outward forms of democracy but not its reality. We may still have elections and political parties but these do not effect real change. That is because effective power lies elsewhere. It lies with those who control the levers of the global market – the multi-national corporations, international financiers and large States. Compassionate activism compels us to challenge and contest this structure in favour of the humanization of all through a commitment to dialogic practice.

CHAPTER NINE

Conclusion: Compassionate Activism

The previous chapter presented a working methodology for integral social care practice. In this concluding final chapter, in order to make tangible the values and principles outlined above, we shall further examine the implications and meaning of dialogic practice for both professional carers and compassionate activists generally. First, we will briefly focus once again on the person who we encounter in integral social care relationships so as to address the importance of the ethical framework which should guide those relationships. We may be guilty of some repetition of themes but the importance of ethics to our practice warrants further emphasis.

This is in part because social care as a professional practice and as a humanistic responsibility of all citizens has been severely undermined in the last number of decades. As a professional practice it has been undermined by the severe and often cruel resource contractions which have occurred due to States withdrawing more and more from direct social care and welfare provision. This has frequently resulted in carers operating in highly constrained and stressful situations and in service users receiving care services that fall far below what they require. In Ireland particularly, social care has been tarnished by reports and revelations into how we have cared for our young children, our teenagers, those with physical, intellectual and mental disabilities, and our old people. As a humanistic responsibility it has been undermined by ideological structures which frequently paint the 'poor and needy' as personally responsible for their own difficulties, as morally inferior and as little better than spongers and deliberately dependent. A dominant conception of human beings as self-interested rational actors who should provide for their own needs has given us a picture of ourselves that elevates private consumption to be the purpose and goal of the rational and good life.

It is beyond the scope of this book to examine all of this. However, the book has attempted to challenge the assumptions underlying these ideas and has argued that care and compassion are in fact inherent and defining aspects of our humanity and that integral social care can be revitalized as an exciting and radical project of human liberation. Committing ourselves to humanization benefits all of us. It is an utterly false notion that each of us can exist in solitary well-being while disregarding the suffering of others. Real self-interest lies in a harmonious, peaceful and equitable society and world.

At the conclusion of this book, I think it may be helpful to restate, even at the risk of revisiting arguments previously made, some of the essential values which may serve as the defining features of an ethical and authentic integral social care practice. These values do not just refer to professional practitioners. They have relevance for all of us as citizens and could indeed constitute the ethical principles of a new humanistic commitment to personal and social well-being. We will outline six core values and then refer briefly to the rich philosophical reflections developed by the philosopher Martin Buber on the centrality and significance of relationships in constituting the purpose and meaning of human existence. We will then conclude by sketching some final features of compassionate activism particularly in its socio-political expression.

Integral social care: a restatement of values

First, the intention of integral social care practice is to enter into relationships with other people that are authentic and liberating. The method of doing so is through non-judgemental acceptance and open dialogue. This is an essential foundation on which to ground our practice because otherwise we may be tempted into a commitment to some abstract notion of 'humanity' rather than to specific, individual human beings. We do not wish for a wooly, ethereal love of all. We require particular engagement with the actual people before us. That is why we have suggested that a commitment to care begins right now, among the people we immediately encounter. Care must begin at home, in our families, in our close relationships and in our extended networks. We do not need to roam the streets for the 'needy' – the people we need to care for are right before us.

Our relationships should be characterized by authenticity and should be orientated towards liberation. Authenticity means that, in our dealings with others, we are who we really are and are not hidden behind a false mask. Authenticity permits our communication to be congruent and better ensures that the other person will hear what we say and that we too will actively listen to them. This acceptance of ourselves permits us to genuinely accept the other too. This mutual acceptance is the first step to integral liberation. The other is freed to be who they are and, in the safe setting of acceptance, can uncover their real selves. Liberation is not just interpersonal. The human being's oppression may also be social and political in its causes and we should participate with them in overcoming these also.

Second, in these relationships we are dealing with a person. We need to be conscious of the deep *presence* of a person, of their dignity and of their inherent value. Just consider the eyes and face of another. Consider the power conveyed by those eyes upon us and how affected we are by the look of another person. We cannot lock eyes with a stranger for more than a few seconds without embarrassment and discomfort. The act even of touching someone's hair is charged with meaning.

There is a fundamental unknowingness and mystery to the other person. Therefore, we judge them and intervene in their lives at our peril. We must be utterly respectful of them and keep in mind the fragility and vulnerability of all of us. It is so easy to do harm to another person. We can do so thoughtlessly, by just having failed to properly pay attention. Never must the other person become an object. Never must they be used by us for our own purposes. We enter into integral social care with restraint and respect, motivated by compassion and proceeding through our dialogic practice.

Third, in integral social care we are most likely dealing with a poor and oppressed person in the sense of these terms used in this book. Often this is a person whose freedom has been curtailed due to physical, mental or social factors. As a result, the person's very humanity may have been reduced and marginalized. They may be alienated from their true selves and from the wider society about them. Yet, no matter what condition they are in, even whether they are comatose or severely brain impaired, they remain a human being. That fundamentally is all we need to know about them. Once we recognize and acknowledge our shared humanity then we are obliged by that fact alone to care.

Fourth, we recognize and affirm the humanity of a person by treating them and addressing them as a human being. If there is to be one sentence that captures and summarizes the purpose and method of integral care then it is that sentence. Yet, consider how radical the implications of that simple sentence actually are if we truly applied it to all of our social relations, to all of our social care policies and practices, and to all of our political decisions. However, that is the project that compassionate activism must commit to. In the previous chapter, we have suggested one simple methodology for social and political decision-making which could transform how we shape our society. Treating someone as a human being through a genuine dialogic practice is a process that begins now.

Fifth, if the purpose and goal of integral social care is to facilitate and enable the other to become a full and free person, the extraordinary thing is that, by assisting in humanizing another, we humanize ourselves. By exercising and generating solidarity, compassion and care we nurture and enhance the humanity in ourselves. We thereby liberate and humanize *each other* by entering into relationships that are characterized by mutuality and exchange. The fact is that human beings influence, affect and make each other. How we are literally shapes how the social world is. The corollary also applies – if we dehumanize the other we dehumanize ourselves and contribute thereby to dehumanizing the world. There can be little genuine happiness and comfort if the cries of the suffering ring all about us.

Finally, the poor and oppressed carry values and challenges that are of extraordinary value. We are used to the idea that the oppressed need to be 'fixed', that they are characterized by deficit and lack, and that value lies only with the successful and the competent. However, the paradox is that the very existence of those who need help inspires and causes the genera-tion of the very care and compassion which are the defining characteristics of an enriched humanity. The oppressed summon us to become our better selves and call on us to finally construct a human civilization. This is why so many who work with the poor, whether they are themselves poor or not, report that they have been enriched and have received far more than they themselves have given. To be an integral social carer is not an act of martyrdom and sacrifice, it is rather a privilege for which we should be grateful.[1]

The philosophy of relation: Martin Buber, 1878–1965

One modern thinker who deeply explored these issues was the Jewish philosopher Martin Buber.[2] His ideas, expressed in philosophical terms, reflect many of the values underlying integral care practice which we have presented in this book and may be of help to us in summarizing and concluding our reflections.

The central tenet of his great work *I and Thou* was that human beings are not isolated subjects but are constituted by their relations with others. There is no 'I' without first there being primary relations between that 'I' and others. These relations can take two forms. First, one can relate to another as an object to be observed and experienced. This Buber designates as 'I-It'. Alternatively, one can enter into a relationship with another that is mutual and reciprocal. This he designates as 'I-Thou' (*Thou* is used here as a translation for the more intimate second person pronoun common

---

1   This is not to deny those awful circumstances where, for example, one's child or elderly relative may have a disability or a condition which not only severely constrains their lives but imposes an extraordinary burden of care on us. Care here should never be carried alone but should be conducted with maximum professional and wider social supports. A culture of care means that the carer too must be cared for.

2   All references cited here are drawn from Buber's most enduring book *I and Thou*. I refer throughout to the reprinted English translation published by T. & T. Clark Ltd, Edinburgh (1984).

to many European languages but no longer found in modern English). For Buber, the 'I' emerges from these relationships. It does not pre-exist them. First, there is either 'I-It' or 'I-Thou' and only then can there be an 'I'. In other words, our sense of self is developed out of the dynamic of our relationships to others.

This is an insight of great importance. In that context, it is clear that *how* we relate to others is of fundamental significance for our own identity and humanity. Buber's claim here that a person is formed by his/her relationships with other persons carries strong echoes of the ideas we encounter in Carl Rogers. Buber's distinction between 'I-It' and 'I-Thou' suggests that there are two fundamental modes of encountering other people. Each of these modes carries differing implications and meaning for the character of human existence. Thus, Buber argues that 'the primary connexion (*sic*) of man with the world of *It* is comprised in *experiencing*, which continually reconstitutes the world, and *using*, which leads the world to its manifold aim, the sustaining, relieving, and equipping of human life' (Buber 1984: 38). However, the development of these necessary functions of experiencing and using comes at the expense of our power and capacity to enter into relation.

For Buber, 'I-Thou' relationships are not characterized or driven by feelings as such. Rather, they are distinguished by mutuality, by reciprocity, by what Buber designates as 'meeting' and by dialogue. 'Meeting' is the full and authentic encounter of one person with another. Buber suggests that 'meetings' are privileged moments in human existence. 'When *Thou* is spoken, the speaker has no thing for his object ... But he takes his stand in relation' (4). Relation is necessarily mutual. 'My *Thou* affects me, as I affect it' (15). The *Thou* is spoken with the whole being. 'I-Thou' moments are privileged because they are 'the door into our existence'. Through the *Thou* a person becomes *I*. Thus, relation is fundamental to us and constitutive of our very selves.

Through the 'I-Thou' relation the human being becomes a person. For Buber 'all real living is meeting.' However, we must be *open* to these extraordinary moments when 'meetings' occur. They can be regarded almost as a grace, as a gift offered to us which we must accept in order for them to happen. Otherwise, they are lost and never occur. That is why we must be attentive to the persons about us. 'Meeting' can occur at any moment if we ensure that we are prepared and available and not closed and withdrawn.

Buber describes care or love as the 'responsibility of an *I* for a *Thou*.' If we accept that this is so, then it may become possible, independently of our feelings as such, to come to love all human beings. These feelings of care or love do not lie in us or in the other person. Care and love lie *between* us, in the relationship that exists if we truly meet the other. The 'between' is the place that we must fill with care and compassion. Thus, love and care are not the results of our introspective personal feelings. Rather they arise as the result of our mutual and reciprocal relationships.

For this reason, Buber argues for the absolute centrality that must be accorded to dialogue in human relationships. In dialogue, the person pays attention to the other and addresses the other with respect and openness.[3] As we have noted above, the alternative to dialogue is monologue, where only one person speaks and does so without reference or response to the word of the other.

In contrast to mutuality and dialogic relationships, hatred is by its nature blind.

> Only a part of a being can be hated. He who sees a whole being and is compelled to reject it is no longer in the kingdom of hate, but is in that of human restriction of the power to say *Thou*. He finds himself unable to say the primary word to the other human being confronting him. This word consistently involves an affirmation of the being addressed. He is therefore compelled to reject either the other or himself. (16)

Buber is arguing here that we can only hate another by choosing not to see all aspects of them. Our hatred focuses in on one feature or characteristic. It is not possible to hate when we see the full human person before us. To hate, we are obliged to reduce the humanity of the other to certain partial facets only. That is why the method of acceptance and dialogic practice is

---

3   Buber, who was Professor of Social Philosophy at the Hebrew University in Jerusalem between 1938 and 1951, had a noble record of campaigning and arguing for dialogue between Israelis and Palestinians and Jews and Arabs. He was a leader of the Ichud (Union) Association which sought reconciliation between Jews and Arabs.

the way to encounter the humanity of the other person. Once we encounter their full humanity, hatred and rejection become almost impossible and care and compassion become the appropriate modes of relating.

Buber argues that the capacity to relate extends to nature and to what he calls 'spiritual beings'. Crucially for Buber, in every *Thou* we address the *Eternal Thou*.

> If you explore the life of things and of conditioned beings you come to the unfathomable, if you deny the life of things and of conditioned beings you stand before nothingness, if you hallow this life you meet the living God. (79)

Buber asserts that there is 'a divine meaning in the life of the world, of man, of human persons, of you and of me' (82). The meeting with God that occurs in our meeting with each other does not happen so that the person may concern themselves with God but 'in order that he may confirm that there is meaning in the world' (115).

Whatever about Buber's ultimate religious conception of human life and the existence of God, his work offers a profound and exhilarating depiction of the centrality of dialogic relationships in constituting human beings. Buber argues that the human person is found and forged in the relationships that one has. Without relationships one is moving through a geometric world of objects and things and can only become an object in turn. The central implication of Buber's reasoning that mutual dialogic relationship is the gateway to becoming a person and that love is the responsibility of an 'I' for a 'Thou' cannot but be that the practice of care and compassion is at the heart of the process of humanization. Integral care is not dependent on our personal introverted feelings or even on our moral qualities. Integral care rather is what emerges between one subject and another by virtue of their shared humanity and mutual presence to each other.

Buber's work provides us with a rich and valuable ethical framework which both guides us in entering into human relationships and assists us in understanding what is at stake in those relationships. Crucially, he teaches us that we must not orientate ourselves around regarding the other person as an object. We may *perforce* be obliged at times to regard other people objectively so that we can organize and co-ordinate work with each other.

But we must not consign other people to the status of an object. As we encounter each person that we meet, we must be open to their subjectivity and the mutuality that necessarily arises in choosing to relate to them.

One may reasonably object that all of this, while noble and worthy in aspiration, is incredibly difficult in practice. That is undoubtedly so. But being difficult does not invalidate it. Nor should the difficulty of it be cited to justify abandoning our efforts. As we have said, integral social care is not for the faint hearted. It is tough and requires real commitment and perseverance. It is an old fallacy to imagine caring people as weak and fey. It is the opposite that is the case.

However, Buber's ultimate grounding of human relationships in an unfolding relationship with God does raise the question of whether integral social care requires or benefits from a spiritual perspective or even from an explicit spirituality of its own. Might we need a sense of the divine in order to be inspired and motivated to really care for each other? Is this the best way by which we can overcome the incredible difficulty of practising care and compassion for all? Need our care practice be grounded within a supernatural or transcendent perspective of understanding the human person?

This is a large and deep question which deserves attention and reflection. However, I cannot see how we could possibly answer that *only* those with a religious framework can practise integral care. Such a position is demonstrably and empirically false. People of all cultures and all times, and of all beliefs and none, have practised care and compassion to extraordinary levels. We have argued above that no culture and no society since the dawn of humanity could have survived without care.

What we do need to help us develop our capacity and willingness to care is a deep humanism that recognizes the dignity and intrinsic value of each human life. Whether that commitment to the good of human beings is grounded in a religious faith is a matter for each individual. Sadly, religious belief has been historically responsible for as much death and destruction as it has care and compassion. Yet, seeing the human person as an image of the divine undoubtedly provides an enriching perspective. The human person is the closest image of the divine that we can create and if we choose to describe ourselves as 'children of God' and consequently as brothers and sisters of each other then what we are doing is simply using our deepest and most somber and mythic language to encapsulate the mystery and value of the human person. If this helps to inspire and motivate integral care then that is a positive outcome. Whether there are in point of fact supernatural and metaphysical realities transcending this earth is a question which is, at a minimum, beyond the scope of this book and assuredly beyond the knowledge and competence of this author!

However, I have suggested above that the traditional great religions are important repositories of human wisdom. They have accumulated insights and experiences over many, many centuries. Their conclusions regarding the dignity of the person and what constitutes the good life should not be dismissed lightly. Their sheer continuity and continued relevance over time indicates that they have provided answers and ways of living that millions of human beings have found worthwhile and fulfilling. Of all the dogmas and creeds, theologies and spiritualities that human kind has constructed, there is little doubt that the most common ethic and principle of all is compassion. In their unique ways, all the religious insight of humanity unites around this one simple but profound teaching – human life should be one of compassion. Not only does compassion lead us to care for each other, it has the capacity to bring fulfillment and happiness for ourselves to such an extent that it may lead us to experience what human cultures have described as the divine or the fundamental meaning of life. At the very least, the ubiquitous nature of this ethic suggests that the practice of compassion is deeply in tune with fundamental human nature. This is the positive image of ourselves that we should reclaim.

Compassionate activism

As we have said throughout, compassionate activism does not just refer to professional social care practitioners. It refers to anyone, whether they are professionals providing social care, citizens or non-citizens who are committed to care and compassion, those receiving formal social care services or simply those in a social care relationship. Compassionate activism describes both a commitment and a practice. It involves saying no to being dehumanized in any way and instead asserting and insisting on our dignity and rights as free human beings. Compassionate activism is about bearing witness to our common humanity and being prepared to pay the price of confronting those powerful and sometimes aggressive forces which curtail and diminish that humanity. As we have suggested in the previous chapter, its appropriate mode and method of proceeding is by dialogic practice.

Being a compassionate activist is not just a tactical strategy. It is a mode and manner of commitment and practice which intrinsically conveys a witness about ourselves, about our values, about our disposition towards our fellow human beings and, perhaps above all, towards our adversaries. We need to think deeply about our adversaries because, given the conflictual nature of human relations, and given the inevitable resistance to change which can be expected, we will be confronted by those who oppose us or who seem to be in our way. However, we need to recognize that, in the long term, we and our adversaries have the same interests. Compassionate activism is an affirmation of our common humanity in the midst of our struggles.

It therefore encompasses not just our actions but our words too. Our words reveal who we are. They reveal our spirit and our dreams. The *means* we use to achieve our social and political objectives tell us about the *goals* we have in mind. They express to others the type of world that we want to bring about. Compassionate activism requires real moral courage because when it is practised its legitimacy and claim to justice is not necessarily recognized or accepted by others. Indeed, it is almost inevitably contested. Moral courage is therefore needed in order to stand up at that time of potential conflict and take your position and stance in the always ambiguous, uncertain, contingent ground of the present. History may ultimately determine who was right but history belongs to the future. Compassionate activism cannot avoid engagement in the mess and circumstance of today. It must do so guided by its adherence to its core values rather than to any claim of foresight or superior knowledge about what is to come.

The compassionate activist is not a perfect person. They are certainly rarely heroes and are not saints. Instead, they are above all human. While there are great exemplars of compassionate activism, figures who inspire us by their courage and effectiveness, almost all compassionate activism is practised in the quiet, mundane, non-public settings of homes and communities. Figures such as Mahatma Gandhi, Martin Luther King, Ken Saro-Wiwa, Dorothy Day, Aung San Su Kyi, Nelson Mandela and the three Nobel Peace prize winners in 2011, Ellen Johnson Sirleaf, Leymah Gbowee and Tawakkul Karman, have shown how, even in the midst of great struggle and suffering, compassionate activists can look beyond the immediate conflicts of the present to the time when the conflict is over and life must be restored. These individuals can serve as valuable exemplars and inspirers of what is possible but compassionate activism is primarily a practice rooted in the ordinary not in the heroic. Often it is women, unknown and unheralded, who carry the greatest responsibility of care for children, family and others in their community.

There is thus much at stake. Humanization cannot be taken for granted. Everywhere and at every time, it must be asserted and defended. For that reason it is so important that, in our caring and campaigning, we must meet each other on the plain of our common humanity. Despite our issues and differences, despite the exigencies and imperatives of our struggles, we forget our common humanity at our peril. The greatest danger of all is that the demands and challenges of our commitment and practice lead us to hatred and antagonism rather than to compassion and harmony.

One of the reasons why this danger might arise is that in our caring practice we may often fail and lose. The individual before us may have rejected us. They may not have received the service they so badly need. We may have proven ineffective in trying to assist them in their liberation from a personal or social oppression. The political change that was needed to finally address an issue may not have been made. Our demands may have been responded to with opposition or indifference. In short, we may frequently experience what it is to be powerless and to be defeated. How we react to this and how we cope with failure are crucial moments which reveal the resilience of our commitment to care. It is in this situation that all of the values that we have outlined in this book now find their moment of truth, their efficacy and their validity. Without a deeply rooted rationale for what we are doing and why, we can go astray and have our own humanity diminished due to despair and 'burn-out'.

The fact is that in integral social care – whether in giving care or receiving it – one can be transformed very easily. One can be reduced and embittered by our experiences of poverty and oppression. We have all seen this happen many times to very good and committed people. It is Yeats who captured this best in his poem 'Meditations in Time of Civil War':

> We had fed the heart on fantasies,
> The heart's grown brutal from the fare,
> More substance in our enmities
> than in our loves

But one can also be humanized and ennobled (if one can use such a word nowadays) by our interpersonal and socio-political activism. Some people become profoundly enriched by these experiences and manage to touch deep personal and human resources that allow them to access a vision and well of compassion that permits them to transcend the immediate issues and problems that they are engaged in and to articulate values and principles that are of universal significance.

We need these standards of compassionate activism today more than ever. This is because we live now in an increasingly brutalized world where images of violence and a tolerance of violence hold sway. We have perfected a form of detached violence where war occurs far away and is largely rendered into a technical affair involving an application of technology. We rarely hear the cries and screams of the victims. Tens of thousands of Iraqis were killed so that 'peace and democracy' could prevail in their country. Their stories are unknown to us. There is thus the callous savagery of indifference. Many of us do not know what is happening about us and many do not really want to know.

We also live in a time of ecological devastation. Global warming is almost certainly underway and mass species extinction occurring all about us. But we have little sense of crisis and little sense that we are witnesses to a systemic dysfunction on a geological scale. Once again, the savagery of indifference holds us in place.

We live in a time where politics is regarded as essentially managerial, requiring the skills of the technocrat and the apparatchik. We seem increasingly unable to imagine and believe that politics could ever be a moral force for bringing about social and ecological change or that it is the arena of public ethics and the potential bearer of new visions of the good life.

Finally, we live in a world of growing ethnic, religious and cultural hatreds and intolerance. A macho fundamentalism seems to have emerged in many cultures. To be 'liberal' or moderate is regarded by many as a weakness, almost as a form of malign naivety. In the erosion of the welfare state and the decline in the State's sense of duty and responsibility to its citizens, in the development of globalization and the shift of power towards private corporations, and in the emergence of a *de facto* post-democracy where decisions are made at levels far beyond the participation of ordinary people, a new social heartlessness and indifference is becoming increasingly institutionalized. The approach of the Chinese government seems to represent the epitome of this new model. What matter democracy and human rights? What really matters is wealth and consumerism. We are witnessing a systematic decline in our sense of the social and in our obligation to social values and ethics.[4]

Yet, all around the world, in every culture and society, this system is contested. We rarely hear these stories. As we have said, compassionate activism is practised in the quiet and mundane spaces of our social world. Of course today, too, we have our exemplary persons who demonstrate the very best in humanization and human commitment. Aung San Suu Kyi who has suffered years of house arrest in Burma and the Dalai Lama exiled in India are two figures who, despite appalling personal suffering, have demonstrated remarkable qualities of resilience, peace and compassion. But for every well-known figure such as these, there are literally millions of others who bravely and quietly commit themselves to bringing about integral social care. In Ireland alone, one cannot help but think especially of

---

4   For an excellent treatment of the decline of the sense of the social see Michael D. Higgins (2006), *Causes for Concern: Irish Politics, Culture and Society*, Dublin: Liberties.

the 100,000 domestic carers who day-in, day-out, care for family members in their own home. These are people whose lives are lived in the service of others, often at great personal sacrifice.

Yet, given that the prevailing system is so flawed what approach should be taken in contesting it? Does the evil of the system permit us to do evil in return? Is everything permitted to us in our actions? The only sensible approach to this question I think is not primarily tactical. It must be moral and ethical. At stake in all our actions is our humanity. That is what we are really struggling for. That is what, despite the features of each specific individual and circumstance, is really at issue. Therefore, the questions that we need to address in guiding our responses to the systemic forms of oppression confronting us must be: are we enhancing our humanity or not? Does our practice make us more human or less? Do we inspire others to enhance their humanity or to degrade it? Are we adding love to the world or hatred? Are we adding peace to the world or conflict? In putting these questions to ourselves and recognizing why they are of importance, I think that it is helpful to remind ourselves again that the great majority of people are fundamentally good and caring and that much of the oppression we see all around us is structural and institutional in nature.

It is for this reason that non-violence, in the widest possible sense of doing no harm, must be the *sine qua non* of the compassionate activist.[5] The integral carer must embrace the principle of non-harm as a fundamental value. Our commitment to non-harm, implicitly contained in our dialogic practice, must extend beyond actions to include our words and attitudes. Crucially, it centres on our disposition towards not just those with whom we are in caring relationships but also with those who might be our adversaries. How shall we relate to them? There will be more to say about this below.

---

5   Of course, in our world today there may be certain extreme and unavoidable situations facing good and caring people where violence, or doing harm to others, may be necessary where no other possible choice is available in order to prevent even greater harm. Where there is no alternative in order to save life – yours or another – it may well be justified. But these are by their nature extraordinary circumstances that we do not seek out.

As we confront the sheer scale and extent of human oppression we perhaps need to inspire ourselves with the thought that our willingness and desire to care confers on us a privilege. It is not a burden that we should bear about us with heaviness and misery. It is a privilege to enter into an authentic and liberating relationship with another person and, in however limited a way, to share their life. It is a privilege to be alive and to be human and to be able to humanize ourselves and others. Above all else therefore, the compassionate activist is distinguished by what they love not by what they hate.

As we conclude this chapter and book, we will outline some of the most important features that characterize what we are choosing to call compassionate activism. Once again, it must be stressed that compassionate activism is understood as a dialogic practice which can be undertaken by everyone and is not just a method for professional practitioners. Indeed, conceptualizing professional care within this wider overarching concept may have the consequence of helping to further revitalize the profession and to allow practitioners to see that they form part of a far wider and exciting project of integral humanization. First, we will suggest three distinct steps that can be followed in setting the scene for a commitment to compassionate activism. Then, finally, we will outline four key principles that must guide compassionate activism's dialogic practice.

Towards a commitment to compassionate activism

When we think of social care we need to think beyond the confines of the interpersonal relationship. Integral care obliges us to consider the socio-political setting within which human relationships occur. In considering this setting, and recognizing that it is constructed and capable of change, the most potent single question we can pose is – what kind of social world enhances human care? The challenge then is to orientate our society to better bring that social world into being. What we are seeking is nothing less than a civilization of care. This amounts to creating a social world which is organized in such a way that it provides for the real and basic needs of all. Focusing in on these needs involves us distinguishing between what is important and what is frankly trivial.

Our real needs are clear and basic. They involve food, shelter, education, acceptance and social inclusion. A caring society and a caring world is one in which all basic needs are met. It is eminently achievable but it requires those who have much to share resources with those who have little. That is a matter of human will.[6] But to generate that, people will need to escape the entrancement of false needs and false mythologies of what constitutes human nature and culture. We are not irrevocably locked into a battle for survival where bad and lazy people rightly suffer and where the ungrateful and spiteful need to be suppressed. We need to escape the confines of our illusions and induced sense of powerlessness and wake up to the social and ecological perils that we are really in. We need instead to recognize the enormous capacities and capabilities available at our hands. To do this requires us to make a series of fundamental realizations and to engage in a number of consequent 'deep actions'.

The first realization is that I as an individual must share this earth with billions of other human beings and other life-forms. The first and most simple action we can undertake arising from this realization is that of *deep seeing*. I need to see that which lies open before me – the world of others. I need to truly see what is happening about me. I need to step out of the artificially constructed safety of my life and see the human reality of those people who dwell on the margins. Their very existence will provide an epistemological reality check. Once I see the full picture of what is about me, I cannot but conclude that all is not well with our shared social world.

The second realization is that all those other human beings and life-forms have inherent value. The second action therefore we can commit to is that of *deep respect* for all. I need to recognize that all that lives has, by virtue of that fact alone, intrinsic value. The only appropriate human response to this richness and diversity of life is one of respect. For me to uphold my

6   Cf Sobrino 2008: 29.

humanity, I cannot willingly disregard or be indifferent to all my fellow beings. Their presence about me challenges me to relate to them.

The third realization is that all those other human beings and life-forms are connected to me. The third action therefore to be undertaken is one of *deep response*. I respond because, by allowing myself to become aware of all those others, I recognize that their existence affects me. I cannot be indifferent to them. I cannot pretend that their condition has no impact on me. I cannot live with my eyes closed and my ears blocked. Were I to do so I would be less than human. Blinded and deafened I would exist in my head, master of a barren, solitary universe. Because they are there, I cannot but be affected by them. Thus, I cannot but enter into a world of relations rather than dwell in a world of objects.

How we choose to relate to other people remains a choice for each individual. There is no prescribed template that all must follow. But once one genuinely begins to relate compassionately to others, a process of transformation and humanization cannot fail to get underway. Where this leads each individual depends on their particular circumstances and commitments. What matters is to be orientated in the right direction, i.e. *towards* other people not *away* from them.

Our renewed civilization of care can be built simply and modestly. It does not really require grand schemes or macro-plans. At the socio-political level, it requires rather a considered political programme designed to provide basic needs for all in each society and throughout the world. A civilization of care is predicated upon the assumption that people are fundamentally good and compassionate and will willingly respond to those that they see in need. A formal global commitment to care would mobilize the vast majority of humanity's deep reserves of care and empathy. In assessing whether such a transformation is achievable or not, there is no reason why we should not choose to believe in humanity rather than to doubt it.

At an interpersonal level all our social actions should be done with the intention of enhancing care and compassion. In the mess and difficulty that is human existence this is of course immensely difficult. But prioritizing the values of care and compassion at a young age, and as an issue that should be central in our school and college curricula, should help. It is an extraordinary sign of our systemic priorities that education in care and compassion are not at the core of what we regard as a full and balanced education. Instead, we seem to value rendering people 'fit for the world' as the primary purpose of our schooling, even when that world is so clearly dysfunctional. It has been argued above that experience and wisdom shows that negative actions lead to negativity, and positive actions to positivity. This is how we can re-construct the world, one small action by one small action, to complement the systemic political transformation that we need. We need to construct for ourselves a new ideal image of the human being, one that centres on compassionate action rather than on celebrity-level consumption.

Defining components of compassionate activism's dialogic practice

We want, finally, to conclude this book by examining four key additional components of what we have designated as dialogic practice. These components are crucial in ensuring that our compassionate activism is truly humanizing in its intent and effect. Gaining a clear and well defined understanding of dialogic practice helps us to identify precisely what it is that we mean by compassionate activism. The concept of compassionate activism implies both that compassion is the purpose of our activism (ends) and that our activism is practised in a compassionate manner (means). Primarily, dialogic practice is characterized by an attitude of non-judgemental acceptance, by empathic listening and understanding of the other person and by facilitating them on their process towards enhanced humanization, a process which humanizes the carer also. The additional components of dialogic practice which we wish to consider now are:[7]

---

7   These principles are drawn from my own and others direct and often difficult personal experiences of campaigning in the contemporary world.

1. Uniting means and ends
2. Moral moderation
3. Attitude to our adversary
4. Witnessing to the truth

Our argument here is that these further components serve to properly guide and orientate dialogic practice so that it remains truly grounded in mutuality, in the fundamental ethic of doing no harm and in the progressive project of enhancing human liberation. In addressing each of these components, we will make a number of references illustrating these themes from the work of Thomas Merton.[8] Merton's steadfast commitment to non-violence and social justice, particularly to ending the war in Vietnam and to Black civil rights, was manifested in a succession of powerful writings throughout the 1960s. These writings on peace and justice constitute a rich written resource and depiction of what compassionate activism might entail.

Uniting means and ends

The central argument of this book has been that integral care should be conceptualized as being about humanization. Crucially, not only is humanization the objective of care, it is also understood as shaping the process of care. We humanize the other person and ourselves by the manner in which we address and deal with them. Our means and ends are thus united and considered as one and the same practice. We certainly cannot force humanization on someone. We cannot sacrifice the other person in order to free them.

---

8   Thomas Merton (1915–1968) was an American Cistercian monk and is widely regarded as the United State's leading spiritual writer of the twentieth century. The citations here are drawn from an anthology of Merton's writings on peace called *The Non-Violent Alternative*.

Sometimes in our interpersonal and socio-political activities we can forget that our ends may be good but our means bad. Or, to put it in a different way, just because our ends are good does not imply that all means are permitted. Our ends cannot be peace while our means are violent. Our cause may be just but it does not permit us to do wrong. We must put limits on the permissible and adhere to those standards. Thus, the integral carer pays great attention to the *process* of care. Indeed, we have argued that the carer can and must take responsibility for the process of care but is not fully responsible for the outcome.

Keeping our means aligned with our ends is crucial to any dialogic practice and project of conscientization. It prevents the integral carer from assuming that they have a privileged, more expert view, one that allows them to better identify the destination and objective of the care relationship. Otherwise, if our minds are solely focused on our objective then getting there is all that counts. How we get there becomes then just a matter of arbitrary tactics.

I think this is a mistaken view. The fact is that our means shape and determine the end we will achieve. If nothing else, that is the lesson of history. If we consider conflicts that become violent, we can readily see how the recourse to violence and forceful means creates its own dynamic. Once it begins the unthinkable can become possible. Violence feeds on violence in an escalating cycle. It almost always leads to an accumulation of anger and hatred which only renders us desensitized to the other person.

> The will to kill and be killed grows out of sacrifices and acts of destruction already performed. As soon as the war has begun, the first dead are there to demand further sacrifices from their companions since they have demonstrated by their example that the objective of the war is such that no price is too high to pay for its attainment. This is the 'sledgehammer argument', the argument of Minerva in Homer: 'You must fight on, for if you now make peace with the enemy, you will offend the dead'. ('The Answer of Minerva', Merton 1980: 147–9)

Thus every act of care and every political campaign in favour of care must be guided by primary values which limit the means we are prepared to use. This involves a voluntary disarming of ourselves, a disarming of our assumptions to superiority, of a desire to win no matter what the price and of our capacity to do harm. Therefore, as we have argued above, one of these primary values must be (with some very rare exceptions) peace-making or, putting it more modestly, the principle of non-harm. In this sense, the integral carer ensures that he/she is not blinded by his/her goal. However worthy and necessary the goal may be, not every means is permissible to achieve it. There are also objectives and concerns greater than our immediate task or concern. The objective of attaining peace and humanization is one. This may mean that we lose in the short-term but we surely gain in the long-term by adding to the sum of goodwill and humanity.

One of the primary justifications for making this assertion is that, as has been suggested before on a number of occasions, our method tells much about the legitimacy and value of our goal. Achieving a demonstrable victory in the short-term may not always be the best outcome if, in so doing, we have lost or compromised principles of greater value. At times of maximum anxiety and emotion, with an oppressed human being before us, attention to values is critical. Our commitment to truth and dialogue is a real force for transformation. People do respond to this. They discern your integrity and commitment by your words and actions. We should never compromise on this because, in simple terms, if we do not act with peace and dignity we cannot be instruments of humanization.

In integral care all our actions and words communicate. They all form part of the dialogic relationship with the other person. They tell the other person about what we want to achieve and who we are. The *Ryan Report* showed us what horrors can occur when carers talk of love and forgiveness but act to physically and emotionally abuse others. Beating a child in order to make them good is a gross violation of any ethical and rational standard of behaviour.

The outcome we want can only be built on the means we use. Engaging in a humanizing, dialogic process, grounded on acceptance, becomes a praxis that in itself creates the individual and society we desire. Means and ends become fused. By saying no to power and force and doing so with dignity and resolve we are already saying yes to mutuality and dialogue and telling others about the world we would build. Bitter means will inevitably lead to bitter outcomes. Moral means lead to moral outcomes.

Moral moderation

However, in speaking of moral means, we need to recognize that the compassionate activist must also avoid the arrogance of assuming a moral superiority. The danger is that with justice on our side we think that we ourselves are just. In addition, even more alarmingly, we think we are justified. Often, in order to inspire ourselves or to mobilize support, we may be tempted to create dichotomies and divide the world into black and white. There are those who are with us and those who are against us. All good is here, all evil there. We see this dynamic in countless campaigns. But this is to forget that we are all human. All the aspects of human character are on 'our' side as they are on 'their's' also. That is why we need to be critical, to be reflective and to continually question ourselves. Groupthink and moralization are some of our greatest dangers. Indeed, this book itself may well have fallen partly into that trap. Because we are 'right' on the issues or the values of importance we conclude that we do not have to critique ourselves or our actions anymore. Being 'right', we become intolerant of those who are 'wrong'. They, after all, have been judged by us to be morally inferior to us and therefore we don't have to engage with them.

As Freire argued, we cannot claim to love humanity if we despise the human beings before us. There can be no abstract love of people if we do not engage with the very people about us. To love an abstraction is to love nothing. In Ireland, we have had our experience of patriots who love 'Ireland' but have contempt for the actual Irish people. In our compassionate activism, our commitment to constant dialogue is fundamental, not only with those who we care for, but also with our 'adversaries'. As the Norwegian philosopher and scholar of Gandhi Arne Naess advises us, there should be maximum encounter with our opponent. Otherwise we turn our opponents, or those who we deem not committed to care, into caricatures and partial beings. As Buber has reminded us, we can only hate part of a person. Maximum dialogue forces us to engage with the whole person and that is an integral part of the humanizing process.

The point is that in our argument and campaigning we should be forthright and direct but not morally superior. Our values give us no license to dispense with common decency and courtesy and with what we might call the universe of conviviality and gentleness. If we are to protest then we must do so with the mind of love and respect and not with one of hatred and anger. If we are ever to break the law then we must recognize that this is a solemn action which breaches the system of rules chosen by the people. We must do so therefore with utmost respect and accept our penalty for so doing as an essential part of the witness we are giving to fundamental truth.

> Here it must be remarked that a holy zeal for the cause of humanity in the abstract may sometimes be mere lovelessness and indifference for concrete and living human beings. When we appeal to the highest and most noble ideals, we are more easily tempted to hate and condemn those who, so we believe, are standing in the way of their realization. ('Blessed are the Meek: The Christian Roots of Nonviolence', Merton 1980: 211)

Attitude to our adversary

Because compassionate activism involves a commitment to human liberation and social transformation, it will inevitably lead to conflict. As remarked above, conflict is an inherent aspect of human sociality. There is a continual battle in the social world for resources, power and status. The gain of some appears to be the loss of others. The demand for integral social care, especially one that extends into the socio-political dimension, will almost always lead to opposition and contestation. Therefore, the compassionate activist must always be prepared for conflict. It is consequently of enormous importance how he/she chooses to regard his/her adversary. Primarily, his/her relation to his/her adversary will be shaped by whether he/she regards him/her as someone to be vanquished or to be converted. If the former, then the ground is set for an escalation in conflict. If the latter, then the ground is set for open dialogue and humanization.

In his/her actions, the compassionate activist must be as concerned with his/her adversary as he/she is with their objectives. Our pursuit of our objectives must not blind us to the people about us, including those who oppose us. The principle of non-harm must apply to them also. The integral carer must meet his/her opponent also on the ground of their common humanity. He/she must treat him/her with utmost respect. The integral carer must never act in a psychologically aggressive manner designed to humiliate or provoke him/her. If compassionate activists have done this then they have degraded other human beings, have degraded themselves, have degraded their issues and have reduced the amount of peace in the world. If so, they have themselves defeated their own cause.

That is why in place of antagonism there should be constant dialogue. This makes our opponent no less our opponent. Antagonism has objective causes which we can never deny or wish away. But that does not prevent us treating him/her as a fellow human being.

> Instead of trying to see the adversary as leverage for one's own effort to realize an ideal, nonviolence seeks only to enter into the dialogue with him in order to attain, together with him, the common good of man ...
>
> A test of our sincerity in the practice of nonviolence is this: are we willing to learn something from the adversary? If a new truth is made known to us by him or through him, will we accept it? ...
>
> The key to nonviolence is the willingness of the nonviolent resister to suffer a certain amount of accidental evil in order to bring about a change of mind in the oppressor and awaken him to personal openness and to dialogue. A nonviolent protest that merely seeks to gain publicity and to show up the oppressor for what he is, without opening his eyes to new values, can be said to be in large part a failure. (Merton 1980: 213, 214 and 217)

Witnessing to the truth

Finally, everything that the compassionate activist does in their dialogic practice is centred on his/her witnessing to the final truth that humanization is constituted by freedom and is attained through a reciprocal process of compassion and care. It is to ensure that no word or action on his/her part may impede that truth from being attained that he/she refrains from using all means to achieve his/her ends and that he/she treats even his/her opponent with respect. If we want to assert the ultimate value of compassion, then our compassionate activism is both a witness to that claim and a manifestation of it. By acting compassionately – with care for all others, friend and foe alike – we are bringing compassion and care into the world. Of course we may 'lose' in the short-term and human oppression continue. But we cannot bring about the reign of care by enacting and implementing oppressions of our own. Thus, in all his/her actions and all his/her words, the compassionate activist witnesses to the final truth of humanization. The ethical principles outlined in this book, particularly the principles of non-harm and dialogue, are as much about witness and process as they are about efficacy.

> There is considerable danger of ambiguity in protests that seek mainly to capture the attention of the press and to gain publicity for a cause, being more concerned with their impact upon the public than with the meaning of that impact. Such dissent tends to be at once dramatic and superficial. It may cause a slight commotion, but in a week everything is forgotten – some new shock has occurred in some other area. What is needed is a constructive dissent that recalls people to their senses, makes them think deeply, plants in them a seed of change, and awakens in them the profound need for truth, reason and peace which is implanted in man's nature. Such dissent implies belief in openness of mind and in the possibility of mature exchange of ideas. ('Peace and Protest: A Statement', Merton 1980: 68)

> Non-violence is not for power but for truth. It is not pragmatic but prophetic. It is not aimed at immediate political results, but at the manifestation of fundamental and crucially important truth ... Never was it more necessary to understand the importance of genuine nonviolence as a power for real change because it is aimed not so much at revolution as at conversion. ('Peace and Revolution: A footnote from Ulysses', Merton 1980: 75)

Conclusion

Finally, however, we must once again concede that our claims that care and compassion are the essential constituents of the human person are contestable. They are certainly not provable beyond doubt. For each instance of care and love, we can undoubtedly find another of oppression and hatred. That is indeed the case. Our point has rather been that human beings can choose between possible practices and therefore can choose to construct, however ambivalently and slowly, a civilization of care. Because we *can* do it we *ought*. This is simply because it is demonstrable (this, at least, we can 'prove') that human beings are happier and more fulfilled in a setting of love and care than they are in one of threat and hatred. As we said at the beginning of this book, who after all would willingly choose to dwell in the camps. If we want to live in a civilization of care that extends from the interpersonal to the socio-political dimensions, then we can orientate ourselves to bring it about.

Hence, the image we have employed of the 'compassionate activist' serves as both a description of integral social care conducted by professionals in institutional settings and of citizens in civic settings and also as a normative or an inspiring image of how we human beings can be. In the early twenty-first century, overwhelmed by countless challenges and problems, we badly need a reinvigorated horizon of hope. We badly need to recover our capacity to shape and change the world about us according to the visions and dreams of the social world that we aspire to have. Politics, tarnished and battered, can be reinvigorated to be once again a vehicle that allows us, through argument and dialogue, to construct a world worthy of our highest aspirations. In so doing, the integral social carer commences from the solid ground of the interpersonal, by which his/her authenticity and congruence are established, into the realm of the socio-political where the fundamental values guiding human interaction are created.

The nature of human existence is fragile, interdependent and vulnerable. None of us can survive alone. None of us can afford to remove ourselves from each other. We are tied to each other irrevocably. We are at one and the same time care givers and care receivers. The bonds between us can be tenuous and grudging or they can be strong and secure. We can ensure that the social and psychological space that we all share is characterized by care and compassion rather than by indifference and selfishness. The choice is ours. No one choice can ultimately be 'proven'.

But the way of compassion describes the very best of us. Those who encapsulate it always retain the power to inspire and create compassion in return. The secret to life, happiness and humanization is not that mysterious after all. It lies in simple propositions. That each person should be as free as possible to be themselves. That the basic needs of all should be met. That each moment should be lived mindfully to the full. And that each mindful moment should be filled with compassion for ourselves, for each other and for all life which shares this planet with us. Achieving this, even in part, is the great project and dream of integral social care.

Do we continually fail to live up to these standards? Yes, of course we do. But are we depicting the unrealizable? I think not. At the end of the well-known film *The Mission* the final scene features a brief conversation between the Portuguese ambassador in eighteenth-century South America and the Cardinal sent from Rome to adjudicate on a dispute between the Jesuit religious order and the governments of Spain and Portugal. On behalf of the Pope, the Cardinal has just signed off on the destruction of the Jesuit missions in the centre of that continent thereby causing the death of large numbers of indigenous people and the ongoing destruction of their unique cultures. The ambassador silkily consoles him by saying – 'You had no alternative, your Eminence. We must work in the world. The world is thus.' The Cardinal's anguished reply can serve as both our inspiration and our judgement – 'No, signor Hontor, thus have we made it. Thus have I made it.'

Bibliography

Arnold, B. (2009). *The Irish Gulag. How the State Betrayed its Innocent Children*. Dublin: Gill & Macmillan.

Bakhtin, M. (1984). *Problems of Dostojevskij's poetics: Theory and history of literature* (Vol. 8). Manchester: Manchester University Press.

Balanda, K. and Wilde, J. (2003). *Inequalities in Perceived Health – A Report on the All-Ireland Social Capital & Health Survey*. Dublin: Institute of Public Health.

Beckett, S. (1979). *The Beckett Trilogy*. London: Picador.

—— (1986) *The Complete Dramatic Works*. Boston and London: Faber & Faber.

Berry, T. (1988). *The Dream of the Earth*. San Francisco: Sierra Club Books.

Boff, L. (1982). *St Francis: A model for human liberation*. London: SCM Press.

Brandon, D. (1979). *Zen in the art of helping*. London: Penguin.

Buber, M. (1984). *I and Thou*. Edinburgh, T. & T. Clark Ltd.

Burke, S. (2009). *Irish Apartheid. Healthcare Inequality in Ireland*. Dublin: New Island.

Camus, A. (2002). *The Plague*. London: Penguin Classics.

Chödrön, P. (2001). *When Things Fall Apart: Heart Advice for Difficult Times*. Boston: Shambhala.

Commission to Enquire into Child Abuse Report (The Ryan Report) (2009).

Dalai Lama and Cutler, H. C. (1999). *The Art of Happiness*. London: Hodder & Stoughton.

Davies, B. (2003). 'Death to Critique and Dissent? The Policies and Practices of New Managerialism and of "Evidence-based Practice"', *Gender and Education*, 15:1, 91–103.

Douthwaite, R. (1992). *The Growth Illusion*. Dublin: Lilliput Press.

Edmondson, R. (1984). *Rhetoric in Sociology*. Salem, MA: Salem House Academic Division.

—— (2008). 'Intercultural Rhetoric, Environmental Reasoning and Wise Argument'. In R. Edmondson and H. Rau (eds), *Environmental Argument and Cultural Difference – Locations, Fractures and Deliberations*, pp. 337–64. Bern: Peter Lang AG.

Foucault, M. (1972). 'The discourse on language'. In *The Archaeology of Knowledge*. New York: Pantheon Books.

—— (1988). *Madness and Civilisation. A History of Insanity in the Age of Reason.* Vintage Books.

Fraser, N. (1997). *Justice Interruptus – Critical Reflections on the 'Postsocialist' Condition.* New York: Routledge.

Freire, P. (1972). *Pedagogy of the Oppressed.* London: Penguin Books.

Garavan, M. (2008). 'Problems in Achieving Dialogue: Cultural Misunderstandings in the Corrib Gas Dispute'. In R. Edmondson and H. Rau (eds), *Environmental Argument and Cultural Difference – Locations, Fractures and Deliberations,* pp. 65–92. Bern: Peter Lang AG.

—— (2009). 'Civil society and political argument: how to make sense when no-one is listening'. In D. O Broin and P. Kirby (eds), *Power, dissent and democracy – civil society and the State in Ireland,* pp. 78–91. Dublin: A. & A. Farmar Ltd.

—— (2010). 'Opening up Paulo Freire's Pedagogy of the Oppressed'. In F. Dukelow and O. O'Donovan (eds), *Opening up Classic Texts,* pp. 123–39. Manchester: Manchester University Press.

Grossman, D. (1995). *On Killing: The Psychological Cost of Learning to Kill in War and Society.* Back Bay Books, Little, Brown and Company.

Haight, R. (1985). *An Alternative Vision – An Interpretation of Liberation Theology.* Mahwah, NJ: Paulist Press.

HEAP Report (2009), Tasc and Siptu.

Heidegger, M. (1962). *Being and Time.* New York: Harper & Row.

Higgins, M. D. (2006). *Causes for Concern: Irish Politics, Culture and Society.* Dublin: Liberties.

Holohan, C. (2011). *In Plain Sight – Responding to the Ferns, Ryan, Murphy and Cloyne Reports.* Dublin: Amnesty International.

Klein, N. (2000). *No Logo.* London: Flamingo.

Lovelock, J. (2009). *The Vanishing Face of Gaia – A Final Warning.* London: Allen Lane.

—— (2006). *The Revenge of Gaia.* London: Penguin.

MacGréil, M. (1996). *Prejudice in Ireland Revisited.* Maynooth: Survey and Research Unit, Department of Social Studies, NUI Maynooth.

—— (2011). *Pluralism and Diversity in Ireland – Prejudice and Related issues in early 21st Century Ireland.* Dublin: Columba Press.

Marcuse, H. (1964). *One Dimensional Man.* London: Routledge, and Kegan Paul.

Marx, K. and Engels. F. (1998). *The German Ideology, including Theses on Feuerbach.* New York: Prometheus Books.

Mayo, P. (2009). *Liberating Praxis – Paulo Freire's Legacy for Radical Education and Politics.* Rotterdam: Sense Publishers.

McCann James, C. *et al* (2009). *Social Care Practice in Ireland – an integrated perspective*. Dublin: Gill & Macmillan.

Merton, T. (1980). *The Non-Violent Alternative*. New York: Farrar, Straus, Giroux.

Mollison, B. (1997). *Introduction to Permaculture*. Tasmania: Tagari Publications.

Murdoch, I. (2001). *The Sovereignty of Good*. London: Penguin Classics.

Naess, A. (1989). *Ecology, community and lifestyle*. Cambridge: Cambridge University Press.

O'Brien, J. and Lovett, H. (1999). *Finding a Way Toward Everyday Lives: The Contribution of Person Centered Planning*. Harrisburg, PA: Pennsylvania Office of Mental Retardation.

O'Murchadha, F. (2006) (ed.). *Violence, Victims, Justifications: Philosophical Approaches*. Bern: Peter Lang AG.

Petrini, C. and Padovani, G (2006). *Slow Food Revolution: A New Culture for Dining and Living*. New York: Rizzoli International.

Putnam, R. (2000). *Bowling Alone: The Collapse and Revival of American Community*. New York: Simon & Schuster.

Rancière, J. (1998). *Disagreement: Politics and Philosophy*. University of Minnesota Press.

Ricard, M. (2006). *Happiness: A Guide to Developing Life's Most Important Skill*. New York: Little, Brown and Company.

Rifkin, J. (2006). *The Empathic Civilization – The Rise of Global Consciousness in a World in Crisis*. Cambridge: Polity Press.

Ritzer, G. (2000). *The McDonaldization of Society*. Thousand Oaks, CA: Pine Forge Press.

Robinson, K. S. (2006). *Fifty Degrees Below*. Harper Collins.

Rogers, C. (1967). *On Becoming a Person: A therapist's view of psychotherapy*. London: Constable.

Sartre, J. P. (1956). *Being and Nothingness: An Essay on Phenomenological Ontology*. New York: Philosophical Library.

Schumacher, E. F. (1973). *Small is Beautiful: A Study of Economics as if People Mattered*. London: Abacus.

Seikkula, J. and Arnkil, T. E. (2006). *Dialogical Meetings in Social Networks*. London and New York: Karnac.

Seikkula, J. (2003). 'The Open Dialogue Approach to Acute Psychosis: Its Poetics and Micropolitics', *Family Process*, Vol. 42, No. 3, 2003, 403–18.

—— (2011). 'Becoming Dialogical: Psychotherapy or a Way of Life?', *The Australian and New Zealand Journal of Family Therapy*, Vol. 32 No. 3 2011, 179–93.

Share, P. and Lalor, K. (2009). *Applied Social Care – An Introduction for Irish Students*. Dublin: Gill & Macmillan.

Sobrino, J. (2008). *The Eye of the Needle – No Salvation outside the Poor, A Utopian-Prophetic Essay*. London: Dartman, Longman & Todd.

Stern Review on the Economics of Climate Change (2006), London: HM Treasury.

Wilkinson, R. and Pickett, K. (2009). *The Spirit Level – Why more equal societies almost always do better*. London: Allen Lane.

Wren, M-A. (2003). *Unhealthy State: Anatomy of a Sick Society*. Dublin: New Island.

Index

Rec. Mar.28, 2013